OXFORD MEDICAL PUBLICATIONS

MANAGING ANXIETY

A Training Manual

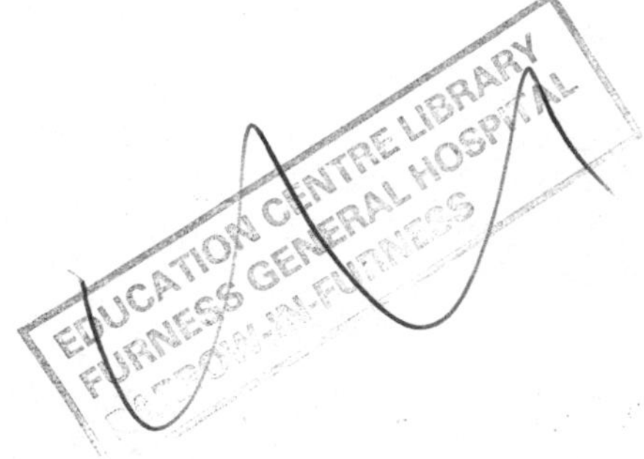

MANAGING ANXIETY

A Training Manual

Second Edition

HELEN KENNERLEY

Department of Clinical Psychology,
Warneford Hospital, Oxford

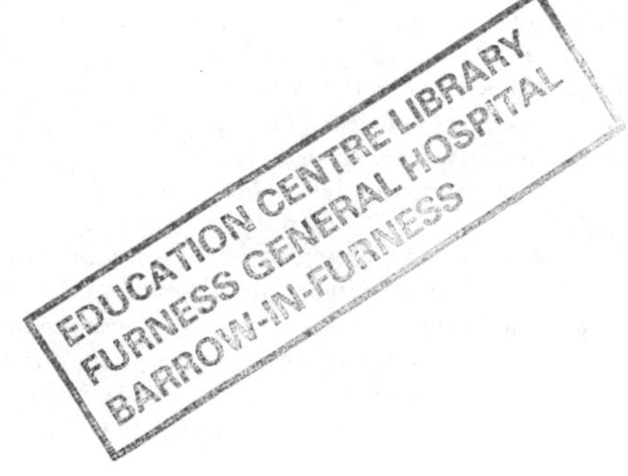

Oxford New York Tokyo
OXFORD UNIVERSITY PRESS
1995

Oxford University Press, Walton Street, Oxford OX2 6DP
Oxford New York Toronto
Delhi Bombay Calcutta Madras Karachi
Kuala Lumpur Singapore Hong Kong Tokyo
Nairobi Dar es Salaam Cape Town
Melbourne Auckland Madrid
and associated companies in
Berlin Ibadan

Oxford is a trade mark of Oxford University Press

Published in the United States
by Oxford University Press Inc., New York

First published 1990
Second edition 1995

A catalogue record for this book is available from the British Library

Library of Congress Cataloging in Publication Data
Kennerley, Helen.
Managing anxiety: a training manual / Helen Kennerley. – 2nd ed.
(Oxford medical publications)
Includes bibliographical references and index.
1. Anxiety. 2. Psychotherapy. 3. Patient education. I. Title. II. Series
[DNLM: 1. Anxiety – therapy. 2. Psychotherapy – methods. WM 172
K36m 1995]
RC531.K46 1995 616.85'2230651–dc20 94-31575
ISBN 0 19 2624423
Typeset by EXPO Holdings, Malaysia
Printed in Great Britain by
Redwood Books, Trowbridge, Wilts

For Hilda and Daisy

Preface to the second edition

Since the first publication of this book, there has been increasing evidence that individuals can learn to manage anxiety with minimal guidance (Marks 1991; Sorby 1991) and that individuals tend to try self-help methods intuitively (Barker *et al.* 1990). Therefore, it is very appropriate that this book is designed to promote self-help and that it contains comprehensive client information sheets to facilitate self-help and improve innate coping methods. The information sheets in this edition have been updated and expanded to provide even more complete guide-lines for suffers of anxiety.

Also, since the first publication of *Managing Anxiety*, Oxford Regional Health Authority provided funding for a further evaluation trial of the treatment outlined in this manual. Feedback from the primary care and psychiatric workers involved in the trial was positive, that is, the manual was again shown to be of practical use to a wide range of community workers. During this trial, requests were made for the updated manual to be broadened to include instruction for helping clients with the anxiety-related problems of post-traumatic stress disorder and 'executive stress' or 'burn out'. Therefore, there are now sections dealing with these problems.

Finally, clients in the trial expressed a desire to learn more about assertiveness and time management. These topics are highly relevant to anxiety management, but are not discussed in detail in this book as they merit training manuals in their own right. However, further supplementary client information sheets on assertiveness and time management have been added to this second edition as an introduction to these important topics.

Oxford H. K.
February 1994

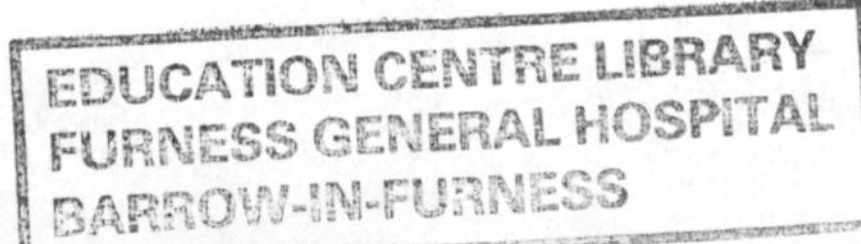

Preface to the first edition

Anxiety-related difficulties are most commonly seen by primary care workers. Every GP has encountered patients with irrational fears, psychosomatic pains, or anxiety induced sleep problems; health visitors are likely to be familiar with mothers of young children who have developed agoraphobia; and the community nurse will almost certainly have come into contact with the anxious relatives of patients who are ill.

Stress-linked problems are also seen by other health care workers who are not based in general practice. Members of psychiatric teams are frequently faced with patients who suffer from fears and phobias concomitant with a psychiatric disorder. Professionals working in general medicine are bound to see patients who have high levels of stress related to illness, investigation, or surgery. Volunteers working in non-statutory organizations that offer support to those with mental or emotional problems meet many people who experience uncomfortable tension in the form of social phobia, agoraphobia, or specific fears. Some psychiatric patients, patients in general hospitals or users of voluntary organizations could benefit from structured therapy to help them cope with anxiety.

This book has been written for health care workers who encounter patients suffering from problem anxiety, and who need to know about the cognitive–behavioural management of anxiety-related problems. Presented here is a psychological approach to anxiety management, which has been compiled to meet the particular needs of non-psychologists. It is intended that this should be a practical guide to anxiety management training, and the contents of this book are divided into three sections.

The book comprises:

- background information: giving the reader the rationale behind the approach;
- preparatory notes for the therapist: to help the user to be thoroughly prepared before starting therapy;

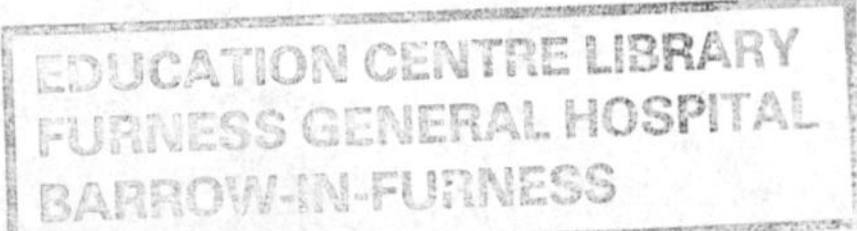

- working with clients: to promote a good working relationship and communication of self-help skills.

Each section is summarized for swift reference once the user is familiar with a technique. There is some repetition across the sections as particular topics are covered for different purposes within each section. This reinforcement of psychological models and techniques will help the user in learning the psychological approach to anxiety management.

The approach set out here is predominantly a behavioural one, with some guidelines for simple cognitive management. Treatment is based in the present and focuses on the individual's current problem behaviours and thoughts, but this is not to deny the relevance of psychodynamic factors in the genesis of problem anxiety. However, working with such issues might not be as appropriate for the non-specialist.

I would like to thank the members of the Department of Psychology at the Warneford Hospital who have been involved both in my training and in providing support while I have been putting together the book, especially Dr John Marzillier who was very encouraging in its early stages. I also wish to thank all the GPs and other health care workers who took part in the validation trial and gave me such valuable feedback on the content of the manual.

Any similarity with real persons in the case histories is coincidental.

Oxford H. K.
1989

Contents

Introduction

Getting started

The following questions are commonly asked by non-psychologists who are considering adopting a psychological approach to anxiety management.

What is anxiety management?

Psychologists are often involved in teaching self-help skills which people can then use to cope in difficult situations. For example, a person might be helped to develop social skills to use in awkward public situations, or may be taught skills for coping with feelings of depression or for dealing with symptoms of anxiety.

Anxiety management training (AMT) was developed by Suinn and Richardson in the early 1970s (Suinn and Richardson 1971). It has proved to be effective in controlling both generalized anxiety and specific fears (Gelder 1985). In its simplest form, the training involves helping someone to identify their symptoms of anxiety and then practise techniques to modify them.

Strictly, the term AMT applies only to the particular approach set out by Suinn and Richardson. However, it is now generally used to describe a structured psychological approach to anxiety management. The techniques which typically make up such a programme are: (1) physical relaxation training, (2) exposure work, and (3) the modification of anxiety provoking thoughts. The goal of therapy is to help the client to develop the personal resources to cope independently with current and future life stresses.

Why use a psychological approach?

In the 1980s, benzodiazepine tranquillizers were the most common treatment for anxiety-related disorders. In Britain, about one in five women and one in 10 men took them at some time. However, there was

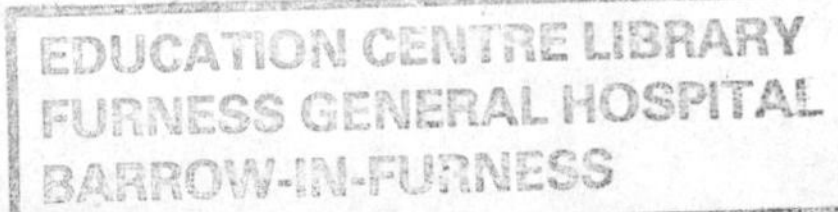

increasing evidence that tranquillizers promoted dependency—sometimes after only a short-term use; that chronic use is associated with adverse effects; and that cessation of use results in a withdrawal syndrome. Further, there were strong indications that drug treatments are no more effective than psychological management (see Catalan and Gath 1985 for a useful review). More recently, Schweizer and Rickels (1991) have shown that benzodiazepines, at best, result in weak and short-lived clinical results. So for some anxiety-related problems, a psychological approach is more desirable than pharmacological intervention.

Why involve primary care workers?

It is estimated that 15 per cent of adults consulting GPs are generally anxious (Lader 1992). This figure is unlikely to include those presenting with specific phobias, discrete panic or obsessional-compulsive disorders, so the prevalence of anxiety disorders in primary care will be considerably greater than this. Minor affective disorders, i.e. anxiety states and/or mild depression, account for a large proportion of consultations in general practice (Goldberg and Huxley 1980). Of these, anxiety is the most common and is most likely to be managed in the practice, rather than being referred on for specialist attention (McPherson 1981).

The primary care worker is, therefore, in contact with the majority of the people who need help in coping with anxiety. Furthermore there are studies which show that such professionals can be highly successful in helping the anxious to overcome their problems by applying psychological methods. Catalan and co-workers (1984) found that GPs can be effective counsellors with patients who would otherwise have been prescribed anxiolytic medication, while Marks (1985) established that trained practice nurses could work well as behaviour therapists in a primary care setting.

Marks (1991) has also established that persons with anxiety disorders, requiring exposure, can benefit from self-administered behavioural treatments. Marks' intervention requires the therapist to assess the problem and then to guide and monitor progress, while the client carries out systematic exposure. The client reports back to the therapist and receives guidance in relapse prevention, but the onus remains on the client to be the active therapeutic agent. Marks concludes that, 'Therapist-accompanied exposure is now known to be largely redundant'. Sorby and co-workers (1991) validated an intervention which required even less professional input. Their study took place in a general practice setting and focused on panic and generalized anxiety disorder. In the experimental group, a self-help booklet was used to supplement the GP's usual therapeutic strategy and proved to be more effective than the GP treatment alone.

There are other good reasons to work at the primary care level. First, the early identification of a problem can improve its outcome. Problem anxiety is most likely to be first presented in general practice, where early intervention is possible. The alternative to beginning therapy at the primary care level is often a lengthy wait for specialist assessment. Secondly, the stigma of attending a specialist service can be avoided. Many individuals have a negative image of a mental hospital and, as a consequence, some are very inhibited about using a hospital-based clinic. This may result in non-attendance for appointments. Thirdly, familiarity with the primary care staff can be a comfort to someone who is being helped through a difficult period. Also, the staff's special knowledge of such a person's background can contribute to a better understanding of the problems and to a more effective treatment plan.

Why involve other non-psychologists?

Health professionals from a variety of settings encounter very anxious or stressed people. Psychiatric workers are regularly dealing with the problem of anxiety, either as a primary disorder or one which is secondary to another emotional problem. Although most psychiatric teams have an association with a clinical psychologist, there are relatively few clinical psychologists in the country, and access to their services is often limited. So, the anxiety management needs of some people are not met unless a non-psychologist can take on the role of therapist. The therapist who already knows an individual through involvement in another role, has often already established a relationship with that person which can then facilitate therapy. Professionals who might take on psychological intervention would be the psychiatric nurse, psychiatrist, psychiatric occupational therapist, psychiatric social worker, or trainee clinical psychologist.

An editorial in *The Lancet* in 1979 concluded that there was evidence of a high prevalence of psychological problems in patients under care in general hospitals, yet the average hospital ward still does not have the support of a clinical psychologist who can advise on the management of stress. The psychological needs of those awaiting surgery, childbirth, or investigation, or those who have specific phobias of hospitals or certain medical procedures, or those recovering from cardiac arrest, might be neglected.

Workers in the voluntary sector try to meet the needs of members of the public who experience emotional problems, but who do not want to seek professional help. The help which is offered is often in the form of individual guidance or group support (relaxation training groups or tranquillizer withdrawal groups, for example). If these public resources are to be effective in helping the person suffering from anxiety, support needs to be properly structured and based on sound psychological principles. Without some form of training or guidance, many volunteers are unable to support some of the people who turn to them for help.

What difficulties might arise?

'*I've already tried a psychological approach without success*'. It is possible that some practice members will have already tried some aspects of anxiety management with their patients; for example, some form of relaxation exercise or exposure might have been suggested. The psychological approach outlined in this manual is a complete treatment programme based on a cognitive—behavioural approach, i.e. one which focuses on the behaviours and thoughts associated with anxiety. It provides a structured approach, aimed at helping people learn coping skills for their problem symptoms. This may be fundamentally different from the approach which you have tried before.

'*I am a GP, I can't fit this sort of treatment into my busy schedule*'. Many primary care workers use AMT successfully. Once problem anxiety has been identified, all that is usually required is one or two extended appointment sessions in order to make a psychological assessment, develop a formulation for the problem, and devise a suitable treatment plan. After this, ordinary sessions are probably sufficient for reviewing progress and offering guidance in homework tasks. This is because the approach is a structured one which depends on the client's doing homework. Although a certain amount of teaching is required, the therapist does not have to give lengthy explanations as all relevant details are given on supplementary sheets for the client.

'*I don't see clients, I have patients*'. This is an important distinction to make. In psychology, the use of the term 'client' denotes a special relationship in which the person in therapy is viewed as a working partner and the therapist as the guide. This active role of the client is distinct from the common impression of a patient, 'a person receiving medical treatment' (*Oxford English Dictionary*). The adoption by the client of a non-passive approach is essential for AMT.

How do I organize this approach?

The user will be guided through a structured approach to managing anxiety, which will involve the following steps:

Identify the problem
If this is anxiety-related

Carry out a psychological assessment
Collect sufficient information to

Formulate the problem
Use this to

Verify the problem with the client
and to

Develop a personal intervention plan
It is also necessary to:

Educate your client about AMT
Then you can begin to

Intervene collaboratively, teaching relevant psychological methods
Guide and monitor progress
Use difficulties or set-backs to

Introduce relapse prevention

As therapy progresses, you will transfer more responsibility to the client.

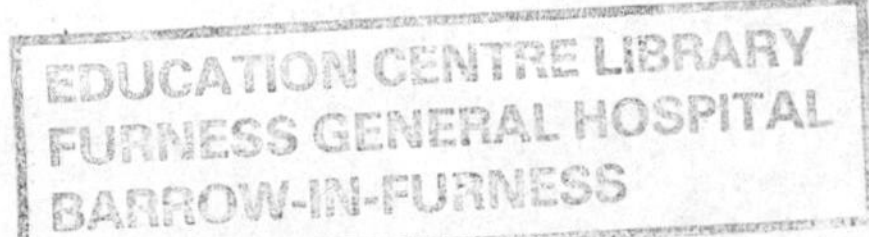

PART I

Background information

1 *Anxiety*

Introduction

Anxiety neuroses are defined as 'various combinations of physical and mental manifestations of anxiety, not attributable to real danger and occurring either in attacks or as a persistent state' (Gelder *et al.* 1989).

There is no simple theory of the development of problem anxiety. The earliest view is based on a psychodynamic understanding of the disorder. The word 'anxiety' entered our language as a translation of Freud's *'angst'*, which was his description of a combination of negative affect and physiological arousal. Neurotic anxiety was viewed as a manifestation of conflicts in the unconscious (Freud 1926). Later, learning theorists suggested that anxiety is not a trait or personality characteristic, but is acquired through classical, operant, or vicarious learning and may develop as a result of real environmental danger or perceived danger (see Marks (1987) for a thorough review). Anxiety states are also associated with stressful external events, particularly those which are interpreted as threatening (Finlay-Jones and Brown 1981). In addition, the finding that problem anxiety is more common among relatives of people who have anxiety neuroses themselves than in the general population (Noyes *et al.* 1978) might support the theory of a genetic basis in the development of problem anxiety.

Clearly, these ideas are not incompatible. Although anxiety can be a reflection of internal states, such as general worries, it is also commonly associated with stressful events and some people do seem to be more vulnerable than others. In assessing an individual, it is important to review all possible aetiological factors.

The development of anxiety

Anxiety is normal and is experienced by everyone at some time. It is an essential response to stress, preparing the individual for action in the face of danger. There are many occasions when the response is reasonable or even vital.

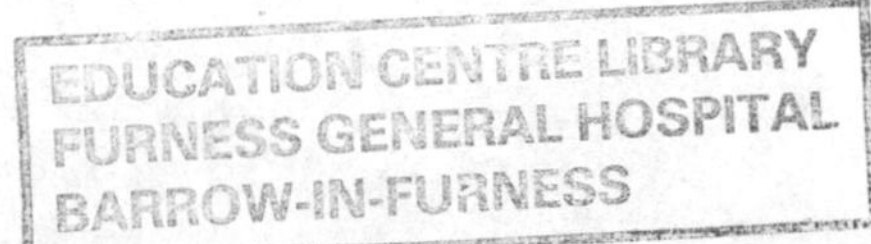

When there is real stress or danger, the body prepares itself for action by releasing adrenalin and the bodily sensations of anxiety become apparent. At these times, the stress response may facilitate physical and psychological performance, but beyond a certain point, functioning is impaired. For example, the body is perfectly prepared for flight and/or fight when adrenalin triggers a surge in blood supply to the muscles, an increasing muscular tension, an increase in respiration and heart rate, and sweating to cool the body. However, when blood is diverted from the skin, paraesthesia can result; protracted muscle tension gives rise to pain; increased breathing can cause hyperventilation; a pounding heart can be alarming, as can marked sweating. A person who is worried by the physiological response to stress can be disabled rather than enabled. Similarly, psychological changes occur in response to stress and we become alert and focused, which is to our advantage when we have to think quickly and cannot afford to be distracted. The psychological stress response is counter-productive when alertness develops into hypersensitivity and chronic worrying. This, in turn, impairs concentration and memory. The benefits and disadvantages of arousal are illustrated in the stress and performance curve shown in Fig. 1.1.

Anxiety influences many aspects of human functioning from perceptual ability, learning, and memory to appetite, sexual functioning, and sleep. Problem anxiety can impair a wide range of abilities and manifest itself in many different forms.

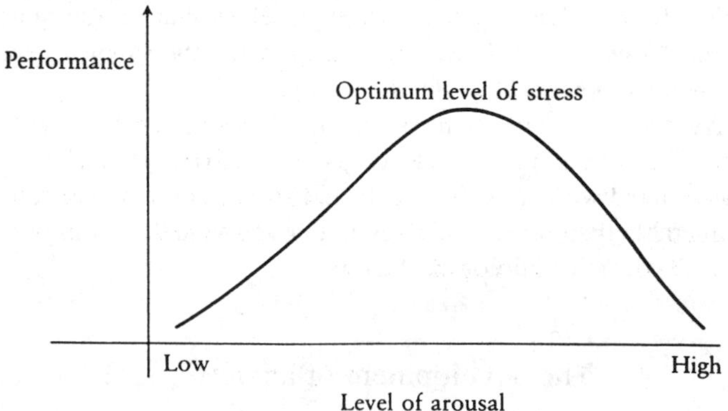

Fig. 1.1 The stress and performance curve

The development of problem anxiety

The feeling of anxiety is provoked by antecedent stimuli or trigger events. These might be external, for example certain animals, heights, or busy traffic; or internal, such as a sudden worrying thought. Often there is a combination of external and internal events leading to the painful sensation of angst.

The natural stress response evolves into a problem stress response when it triggers a cycle of distress. If a man was threatened by a dog in the street and he became extremely panicky, his immediate behaviour might be to rush to his car and leave the area. This action could so undermine his confidence about coping in a similar situation that he might begin to avoid going into the street at all. The long-term consequence of this could be agoraphobia. The immediate response of a woman who had a panic attack while shopping in a supermarket might be to escape from the shop. The trauma of the panic attack could trigger a fear of it happening again, and she might then take a tranquillizer to enable her to cope with shopping. The long-term consequence of this could be the development of drug dependence. The result of such responses to fear is the development of maintaining cycles of anxiety and distress, which can continue in the absence of a stressor or which grows out of proportion to its cause (see Fig. 1.2).

The most common consequence of anxiety is avoidance of the feared object or situation. Unfortunately, the relief afforded by avoidance is only temporary and if avoidance becomes habitual, the object or situation becomes increasingly difficult to face. By never confronting a fear, the sufferer never learns that the object may be benign and so the fear persists. A result of persistent fear is the development of a cycle of anxiety which exacerbates the stress further.

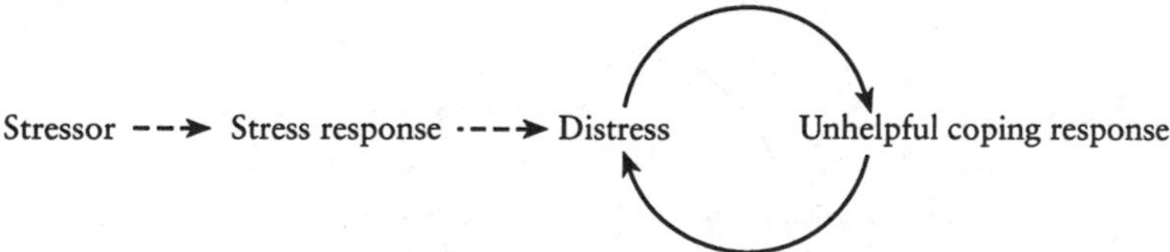

Fig. 1.2 The cycle of anxiety

Avoidance maintaining anxiety

Avoidance can present in an overt form: someone's never going into large shops, never driving, never speaking in public, for example. Avoidance can also be practised in more subtle ways which are harder for the therapist to detect.

A client might seem to be facing a fearful situation, but is relying on a 'crutch' to get them through. This is often in the form of alcohol or tranquillizers, but can be even less obvious. I worked with a client with health fears who seemed to be quite able to travel around the country—it transpired that he could do this only because he carried a mobile telephone and the numbers of local hospitals. Another client was, apparently, able to go shopping despite her agoraphobia—this was because she pushed a baby buggy in front of her which lessened her fear that she would collapse. Other clients use friends, rituals, supermarket trolleys, or a talisman in order to avoid facing what frightens them. Someone who attends difficult situations but then escapes from them is not only practising avoidance, but actively confirming that she or he cannot cope.

Other maintaining cycles

Fear of fear

The physical experience of anxiety and worrying thoughts is frightening and thus concomitant with increased tension. This further exacerbates the physical symptoms and/or the worrying thoughts, and a cycle develops. This is the beginning of problem anxiety—anxiety which can continue in the absence of a stressor or which grows out of proportion to its cause. Anxious people eventually begin to anticipate this unpleasant anxiety response, which can in itself cause anxiety. This is the fear of fear response, shown in Fig. 1.3.

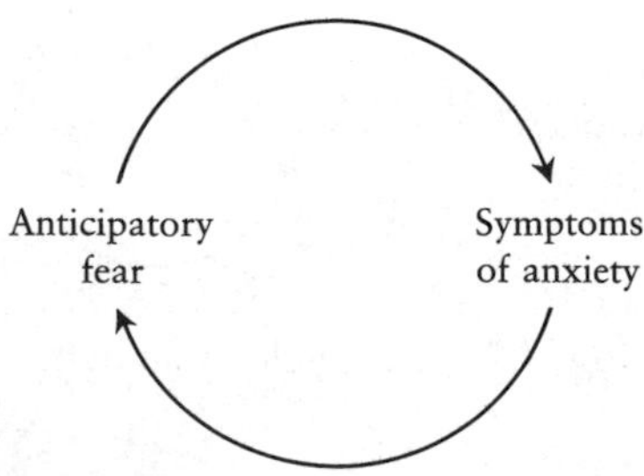

Fig. 1.3 The fear of fear cycle

Short-term reinforcement

Many immediate responses to distress give swift relief which does not, necessarily, last. The manager who turns to heavy drinking in the bar after work does not solve his business crisis and almost certainly impairs his ability to problem solve and plan. The issue is there the next day and if, again, he copes with the stress by using alcohol, the problem may worsen. The person with hypochondriasis gains immediate relief by consulting the GP but, within hours of reassurance seeking, is again worrying about illness because he has not developed the confidence to assure himself. Avoidance is another example of short-term coping which undermines long-term stress management.

Catastrophic misinterpretation or prediction

This is a common maintaining factor in panic disorder. Typically, a person experiences a physical sensation which is benign and misinterprets this as threatening to life, sanity or self-esteem. Chest pain triggered by indigestion becomes a heart attack; a tension headache becomes a brain tumour; the symptoms of hyperventilation are thought to indicate madness; light-headedness is interpreted as impending collapse and humiliation. Events also trigger catastrophization: a routine job review is assumed to herald redundancy; news that one's son and wife are about to drive from Scotland to London triggers images of motorway crashes and his children being orphaned.

Hyperventilation or overbreathing

Hyperventilation is a consequence of heightened arousal and thus a common corollary of anxiety and panic. It causes alkalosis (over-oxygenating of the blood) which gives rise to physical symptoms such as: dizziness, tachycardia, palpitations, blurred vision, paraesthesia, nausea, and breathlessness. These symptoms can easily be misinterpreted as the symptoms of fear, of physical illness or of mental illness and can, thus, maintain anxiety.

Thinking bias or cognitive distortions

When any of us is anxious, we are more prone to cognitive distortion. Weeks before a stressful event, such as an exam, we might be optimistic and sanguine, but as the event nears, our anxiety rises, optimism deteriorates and we can lose objectivity. Typical thinking errors at times of high anxiety are: dichotomizing (only seeing 'black' and 'white' categories, not appreciating the 'grey' areas) and then overgeneralizing from the negative. This might be compounded by an inability to acknowledge any positive events at all. Jumping to negative conclusions on the basis of 'mind reading' or intuition is also more likely to occur under stress, as is self-blame. Clearly, the more negative the thinking process the more likely is the exacerbation of stress which then fuels negative thinking.

Scanning or hypersensitivity

It is not uncommon for a client, who is afraid of something, to search for it. The person with a spider phobia keeps a constant watch for spiders or webs, or cracks in the wall which could house a spider; and the individual with cancer fears repeatedly checks and feels their body for signs. The consequences of these actions to restimulate the fear: if there is present a cause for concern, it is never overlooked. On the other hand, if there is an ambiguous stimulus, it tends to be perceived as threatening—a bit of fluff on the carpet is seen as a spider; a harmless nodule under the skin is believed to be cancerous.

Performance anxieties

Predicting that the worst will happen can undermine confidence and precipitate failure. For example, if I believe that I will spill tea into a saucer as I carry a drink across the room, I will probably be so tense as to spill it; if a student predicts that he will forget his subject during an exam, his nervousness is likely to impair his recall; someone who is certain that she will have diarrhoea during a car journey could worry herself enough to cause the condition. The individual's stress-related response then confirms the belief, 'I can't do X'; this belief strengthens negative predictions in the future.

Systemic maintaining factors

Not all maintaining factors are internal. Sometimes problem anxieties are perpetuated by a stressful work or home life, or by reinforcement by others. The husband who responds to his wife's pleas to reassure her about her health; the helpful neighbour who does not mind always fetching his agoraphobic friend's shopping; the older brother who taunts his phobic sister and thus diminishes her confidence further, all collude in maintaining an anxiety-related problem.

At this stage, problem anxiety can be maintained in the absence of an actual stressor.

What to look for: symptoms

Anxiety has three components: behavioural factors, physical symptoms, and worrying thoughts.

Behavioural factors

Anxiety can directly affect behaviour and impair performance. For example, it can cause stuttering, insomnia, hypermobility, and repetitive behaviours. By far the most common behavioural disturbance is avoidance or escape.

Physical symptoms

Over-activity of the sympathetic nervous system or increased muscular tension is experienced in the form of a variety of bodily responses for which the sufferer might seek medical help.

Common respiratory symptoms include feelings of constriction in the chest, difficulty in inhaling, and overbreathing, while cardiovascular consequences are palpitations, discomfort or pain over the heart, and throbbing in the neck. Complaints relating to the central nervous system include tinnitus, blurring of vision, prickling sensations, and dizziness.

Symptoms related to the gastrointestinal tract include dry mouth, swallowing difficulties, epigastric discomfort, flatulence, and frequent or loose motions. Genito-urinary symptoms may include increased frequency and urgency of micturition, impotence in men, loss of libido, and complaints of amenorrhoea or dysmenorrhoea in women.

Other symptoms may relate to muscular tension. In the scalp this is felt as headache, usually bilateral and in the form of a pressure headache. Tension in other muscles may be experienced as aching or stiffness and hands may tremble. A probable sequel to muscular tension is fatigue.

Worrying thoughts

These are distressing and often repetitive thoughts which accompany increased arousal. Such thoughts or fantasies concern the possible danger of external physical threat, but are more often fears of psychological or physiological harm. For example, someone in an aeroplane might constantly worry that it will crash; an individual in a crowded shop might fear that they will collapse and look foolish; a person who is panicking might misinterpret this as the onset of physical or mental illness. Such worries are frequently provoked by awareness of physical tension, which is then prolonged by the worrying thoughts.

Worries need not always be in the form of words, although the client will have to learn how to express them verbally. Post-traumatic flashbacks are cognitive symptoms of anxiety wherein an event is 'replayed' in imagination. This is involuntary, distressing, and sometimes so realistic that the person believes that the situation is being relived. Some worrying thoughts are self-generated alarming images ranging from realistic to very bizarre pictures. As these are stored as non-verbal experiences and because the image might be strange, clients often have difficulty sharing them and need much encouragement. Some worries are not even in the form of pictures but are automatic, physical reactions. For example, a person's response to seeing a spider might be a shudder, without words or pictures. In time, she or he might be able to express this as, 'the sensation of a spider crawling in my hair—that's what I fear most of all'.

It is also important to note that excessive anxiety can effect other cognitive changes, as it impairs concentration and memory. People find themselves less able to attend to, and to recall information, which can cause worry about work performance or fear of dementia, and this in turn worsens the original anxiety.

To sum up, these three components are likely to be present in combination, with variation in the extent to which each is manifested (Fig. 1.4). It is important to consider all three aspects when assessing anxiety.

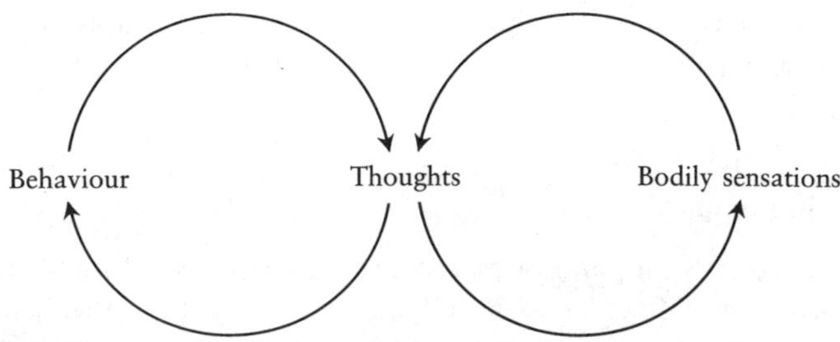

Fig. 1.4 The interaction of the three components of anxiety

The individual concerned might have already identifie as anxiety, but this is not always the case. An anxious well present with the physical symptoms of stress rather for anxiety itself. Therefore, the condition can be mistaken illness, especially if the client is unwilling to acknowledge a psychological problem. The correct diagnosis depends upon finding other symptoms of anxiety and asking about the order in which the symptoms are experienced during an attack. In a paroxysmal tachycardia, for example, it should be ascertained whether the awareness of rapid heart action comes before or after the feeling of anxiety. Further, the conditions that maintain the sensations should be clarified.

Disorders which might be mistaken for anxiety

Anxiety states need to be distinguished from other psychiatric disorders and from physical illness. A degree of anxiety can occur in all psychiatric illnesses but in some instances there are likely to be particular diagnostic difficulties. Anxiety is a common symptom of *depressive illness*, while the syndrome of anxiety neurosis often incorporates some depressive symptoms. The two syndromes can usually be distinguished by the relative severity of symptoms and the order in which they appeared.

Presenting 'anxiety' might mask other problems such as marital disharmony or work troubles, and this possibility should always be explored. *Pre-senile or senile dementias* occasionally come to notice because a person is complaining of anxiety. The clinician might then overlook memory problems, the crucial symptom of dementia, regarding them as the result of poor concentration.

The *effects of drug or alcohol use* may be misinterpreted as symptoms of anxiety. Recording details of the onset of unpleasant symptoms is helpful in establishing a relationship between the symptoms and substance abuse. More commonly, the sensations of *drug withdrawal* are confused with those of anxiety and the use of drugs may be a means of alleviating the effects of withdrawal. Withdrawal symptoms are most likely to occur on waking in the morning. According to Ashton (1984), caffeine is anxiogenic, producing symptoms indistinguishable from anxiety neurosis. These include insomnia, headache, irritability, tremor, nausea, and diarrhoea. Caffeine has been shown to produce tolerance and physical dependence with a withdrawal syndrome of dysphoria, headache, lethargy, irritability, poor concentration, and anxiety. People with panic disorders have been shown to be particularly sensitive to the anxiogenic effects of caffeine.

A useful review of organic causes of anxiety-type symptoms was compiled by McCue and McCue (1984). They drew attention to the following physical conditions. First, the endocrine disorder *thyrotoxicosis (hyperthyroidism)*, which can produce anxiety-type symptoms. This is more likely to occur in women than in men and is most common between the ages of 30 and 60 years. Although many features of anxiety states are present, there are certain differences, i.e. weight loss despite a normal or increased appetite, preference for cold weather, physical signs such as cardiac arrhythmias, tachycardia persisting during sleep, palpable thyroid gland, and exophthalmos. In addition, there is often an absence of a prior history of stress or anxiety.

Secondly, the symptoms and signs of *hypoglycaemia*, or low blood sugar level, which include weakness, sweating, palpitations, tremor, faintness, dizziness, headache, and double vision. These could be misinterpreted as the symptoms of a panic attack. Ascertaining the blood-glucose levels at the time of an 'attack' can help to differentiate the conditions.

Thirdly, episodes of *paroxysmal tachycardia* which can produce symptoms that resemble anxiety—sweating, pallor, faintness, exhaustion. Like anxiety, paroxysmal tachycardia can be precipitated by caffeine, alcohol, and tobacco use. However, the pulse rate is often much faster than in the anxiety state and bouts often occur without precipitants. Where possible, an EEG reading taken during an episode should enable a correct diagnosis to be made.

What to look for: types of anxiety.

Although anxiety neuroses have shared features, there are different categories which are characterized by different presentations. The types you are likely to see are: generalized anxiety disorder (GAD), fears and phobias, panic disorder, obsessive-compulsive disorder, post-traumatic stress disorder (PTSD) and, what is now called 'executive stress' or 'burn out'.

Generalized anxiety

This refers to a persistent and widespread feeling of anxiety which might, at first, seem to be unrelated to specific situations, events, or objects. Beck and co-workers (1985) argue that individuals suffer chronic anxieties because they hold beliefs or assumptions which lead them to interpret a wide range of situations as threatening. Common themes are: competence ('My work is not perfect, therefore it is unacceptable'); acceptability ('I have displeased John and so he will reject me'); self-worth ('I have few friends and few qualifications, I must be worthless'); and control ('If I am not totally in control, I will lose control, and that is dangerous'). Although Beck's model points to discrete triggers of the distress, clients often report feeling anxious 'all of the time' and 'for no apparent reason'. It might be some time before the client can clarify the triggers and the beliefs which explain GAD.

Symptoms of heightened autonomic arousal are experienced, signs of tension are evident, and mild depressive symptoms are common. Frequently the person is apprehensive and has many fears which are likely to relate to the anxiety itself, for example, fear of madness or physical harm. The symptoms of generalized anxiety are similar to those found in other anxiety states but are characterized by their persistent and generalized nature and by the absence of a specific focus.

Often, someone who reports suffering from generalized anxiety will, on examination, be found to be experiencing a specific fear or a number of fears. Care must be taken to tease out each phobia from the collection of fears which may have been described as generalized anxiety. It is also possible that particular phobias are present in combination with generalized anxiety, and this should be considered in an assessment of the problem.

A case of generalized anxiety: Mrs Green

Mrs Green was a 50-year-old, divorced woman who had recently moved to a new village. She attended the surgery of her new GP, asking for help with 'anxiety'. She said that she felt 'constantly on edge, as if something were about to happen', she added, 'I can't rest; I can't sit still or apply myself to anything; I just can't cope'. When her doctor explored further, she described a good deal of physical discomfort: muscular tension, especially in her shoulders, neck, and head; dizziness; blurred vision; shortness of breath; nausea and frequent episodes of choking on food. She was no longer sleeping properly, in that she had difficulty in getting off to sleep and experienced early wakening. Her previous GP had given her a thorough physical investigation and had established that her symptoms were not organic in origin. Mrs Green was quite satisfied that her symptoms were of anxiety.

The GP asked Mrs Green what sort of thoughts ran through her mind when she felt so physically uncomfortable. She replied that she anticipated the feelings worsening to the point where she would collapse. She believed that she would never be free of these awful sensations. She added that the more she thought about the sensations, the worse they became. Her worrying thoughts were especially troublesome when she was alone or when she was feeling ill or miserable.

When asked what she did in order to relieve her condition, she said that she tended to take one of the tranquillizers which her previous doctor had prescribed, or she smoked a cigarette. In fact, the number of cigarettes which she smoked had risen from three to 25 a day over the last two years. She had also begun to avoid going out, in case her fear of collapse was realized and she would embarrass herself. However, she was willing to venture out with the support of someone else, or at night when she felt that no one would witness her distress.

Her GP wondered just how long this had been a problem and Mrs Green said that this constant feeling of tension began about two years ago, although she described herself as being 'an anxious person'. Her greatest fear now was of 'becoming agoraphobic, like my mother' and this is what had led her to seek help.

Fears and phobias

Mild fears are common but become a problem when the feelings are abnormally intense and lead to the avoidance of certain objects or situations. The fear is recognized by the sufferer as excessive or unreasonable in proportion to the actual dangerousness of the object or situation. The phobic response is generally heightened during periods of stress, illness, and particularly depressed mood. Three main phobic syndromes are recognized: simple phobia, agoraphobia, and social phobia. The first two phobias are more common in women, social phobia being equally common in both sexes.

Simple phobia is the irrational fear of a specific object or situation. The fear is often discrete and the sufferer free of anxiety symptoms unless faced with, or anticipating, the phobic stimulus. The most common simple phobias involve animals, especially dogs, snakes, insects, and mice. Other common fears are claustrophobia (fear of closed spaces) and acrophobia (fear of heights). Historically, phobias were classified by the name of the object of fear, which has given rise to an exotic nomenclature: for example, anthrophobia (fear of flowers), ailurophobia (fear of cats), brontophobia (fear of thunder), and ophidophobia (fear of snakes). Whatever the source of the fear, the condition has three components: the typical somatic symptoms of anxiety, anticipatory thoughts, and avoidance of the fear-provoking stimulus.

Agoraphobia literally means 'fear of the market-place'. In practice, it is used to describe a fear of being alone, or of being somewhere from which escape might be difficult, or a fear of leaving a place of safety, usually the home. The symptoms are so diverse that it has been suggested that agoraphobia is not a single syndrome. However, a central group of symptoms can be identified. The somatic sensations are similar to any anxiety state, while the associated anxious thoughts are characteristically centred on ideas of fainting, physical harm, or losing control. The situations in which symptoms appear tend to be those which hinder escape, such as public transport, busy shops, or lifts. A pattern of avoidance develops and the condition may progress to the extent that the person becomes wholly housebound. Agoraphobia might occur with or without panic attacks and incorporate one or more phobias.

Social phobia is the fear and subsequent avoidance of situations where one might be observed or exposed to the scrutiny of others. The phobia might take the form of a fear of writing in public, of meeting strangers, or of public speaking, for example. The socially phobic person typically believes that others notice the symptoms and make evaluations accordingly. This then increases his or her tension. Marked anticipatory anxiety is a feature of social phobia and it often leads to some form of avoidance. Tranquillizers and alcohol may be taken as a means of avoiding the unpleasant sensations and cognitions of anxiety and it is of note that alcohol abuse is more common in this phobia than in the other phobic syndromes.

A case of simple phobia: Mrs Smith

Mrs Smith was a 30-year-old mother of three, who was happily married to a lorry driver who worked away from home a good deal of the time. Her particular problem was identified by her health visitor on a routine visit to see the 12-month-old baby.

During the visit, Mrs Smith suddenly gasped with fear as a wasp crawled from behind the curtain. She went pale and began to shake, saying that she felt sick and had to get out of the living room. She raced into the kitchen, and after the health visitor had managed to get rid of the wasp, they sat down to talk about the incident. Mrs Smith refused to return to the living room, and they stayed in the kitchen to discuss the incident.

It seemed that she had suffered from a wasp phobia for several years, but this had become more marked in the last 18 months. Whenever she saw a wasp, or even suspected that one might be near by, she experienced the physical symptoms witnessed by the health visitor and would run from the situation. She also took 'anti-wasp' precautions from April until November, such as always keeping windows closed, never shopping at the local greengrocer's, which had fruit on open display, never allowing her children to eat sweets outside in case this attracted wasps, and she had bought a tumble drier so that she would not have to peg out the washing in the garden. In fact, she had not been in her own garden during the day for the past two summers.

Interestingly, she was not afraid of being stung by a wasp, but that one might touch her. The mental image which was evoked when she saw a wasp or believed one to be nearby, was of the insect crawling on her or caught in her hair. This immediately made her skin tingle and she felt sick; indeed, she experienced nausea just talking about it. She was also fearful of bees and spiders, but to a lesser extent as she perceived them as less likely to crawl on her.

Episodes of acute anxiety lasted only a few minutes, although she was always uneasy when out of doors in the summer, or when she anticipated having to go out of doors. In all other respects, she described herself as quite relaxed and generally happy. When the health visitor asked her what she believed was happening when she felt so awful, Mrs Smith was reluctant to answer. Eventually she was able to say that she thought that she must be going mad and that these episodes were the early stages of insanity.

Panic attack

A panic attack comprises an intense feeling of apprehension or of impending disaster which is of sudden onset and associated with a wide range of distressing physical sensations. Hyperventilation and alkalosis are common in panic attacks and fuel escalating panic by triggering dizziness, vertigo, tachycardia, palpitations, blurred vision, paraesthesia, nausea, and breathlessness. During an attack, a person fears that something very alarming is happening, such as a heart attack, a stroke, or madness. The experience usually lasts for only a few minutes and is intensely unpleasant. The majority of panic attacks is preceded by bodily sensations and terror results from the catastrophic misinterpretation of these feelings. The sensations which are misinterpreted are those usually associated with anxiety. The sufferer often develops varying degrees of nervousness and apprehension between attacks.

Panic attacks may occur as part of another anxiety problem. For example, some people with agoraphobia have experienced a panic attack and this has made them fearful of repeated attacks when away from a safe base.

A case of panic attack: Mr Peters

Mr Peters was a successful, 40-year-old businessman who had begun to consult his GP very regularly in order to check his health. His first appearance at the surgery followed a series of unpleasant incidents in his car. He described a recent episode as follows: 'I was driving back from a business trip 50 miles away when I got a knot in my stomach, my arms, legs, and lips tingled, my heart was thumping, I began to sweat and couldn't catch my breath. I stopped the car on the hard shoulder of the motorway and was convinced that I was having a heart attack. I could only think how awful it would be to collapse so far from home or a hospital.'

His doctor carried out a physical investigation, was satisfied that Mr Peters had experienced a panic attack and she prescribed Lorazepam. Mr Peters did not find this helpful and became even more convinced that his symptoms must be those of a heart attack and not those of tension. The fact that he did not have a heart attack during these unpleasant episodes did not reassure him that he was healthy. He firmly believed that 'I've got away with it this time—the chance of my having a heart attack must now be greater.' He began to plan all his car journeys so that he always knew how to get to the local hospital. He grew increasingly anxious and he started to have panic attacks whenever he was away from home. When possible, he took his wife or a work colleague with him in the car, which reduced his anxiety slightly. He also arranged to have a lengthy private medical investigation. This again showed no physical abnormality, but Mr Peters was not wholly reassured by this, and returned to his GP.

Obsessive–compulsive behaviours

These are relatively uncommon states defined by subjective feelings of compulsion to carry out an act or dwell on a thought.

Obsessional thoughts and doubts are intrusive, repetitive thoughts or images which are recognized as being self-generated and abhorrent or senseless but none the less difficult to dismiss. The triggers for obsessional thoughts are varied and include thinking or reading an unacceptable word, a certain look from another person, an act—such as using a public lavatory—which runs the risk of contamination. Obsessions cause distress and often provoke compulsive behaviours to ameliorate the powerful discomfort. Unlike preoccupations, obsessions produce much distress. Obsessional impulses and rituals or compulsive behaviours are irresistibly strong urges to perform inappropriate actions. These are stereotyped and performed according to a set of rules in order to neutralize an obsessional thought. The most common compulsive behaviours are cleaning and checking. A mother who worries that she might contaminate and kill her children, because her personal hygiene is not rigorous enough, might neutralize her fears by ritualistic washing. A man whose health fears are triggered by his reading or hearing the word 'cancer' might allay his fears by systematically checking his body for an hour. The compulsive or neutralizing act can be carried out mentally as well as, or instead of, behaviourally and the most likely mental acts are of restitution. The mother described above might be able to allay her fears by chanting her children's names in a certain way in order to confer safety; the man with the cancer fears might be able to think of 'healthy' words to neutralize the trigger word. Anxiety is temporarily decreased by the ritualistic acts, but, in the longer term, anxiety is usually increased by them. The most characteristic sequence is for an obsession to lead to a compulsion.

Obsessional thoughts and compulsive rituals may be provoked in certain situations and it is likely that the individual will avoid such situations. For example, the hygiene conscious mother might bathe five times a day and wear many pairs of disposable rubber gloves in order to avoid feeling unclean, while the health obsessed man might refuse to read books and papers in order to avoid seeing the word 'cancer'. As with other anxiety disorders, avoidance serves to maintain the problem. Anxiety is sometimes decreased by the ritualistic behaviours, but it may also be increased by them. The person who suffers from obsessions is often depressed and symptoms are exacerbated if the depression deepens.

A case of obsessional compulsive behavior: Mr Oldham

Mr Oldham was a 64-year-old administrator for a large business who had gone to his GP complaining of memory problems, which had been worsening over the last year. His fear was that he had developed a dementia. His doctor had arranged for him to have a neurological assessment which indicated that there was no organic impairment. Therefore, his GP began to explore the problem again, asking Mr Oldham to tell him once more what had led him to worry about his memory.

Mr Oldham said that he repeatedly checked that he had carried out safety precautions around the house and at work. It turned out that this was not because he had no recollection of doing something, but because he felt that 'I cannot believe my own eyes and I have to return to check' and, 'If I leave something unlocked or switched on, terrible things could happen'. In fact, Mr Oldham was preoccupied with the terrible things which might occur, such as explosions, burglary, or fire. His thoughts concerned possible catastrophe for more than half his waking time. If he tried to resist the urge to check, he began to feel shaky, his heartbeat increased and he was aware of muscular tension.

He would feel compelled to check things at least three times, but often more frequently. He rarely went back to look more than 10 times, but his safety checks might well involve his getting up several times during the night or breaking his train journey to work. His GP asked if this compulsion was made worse under different circumstances. Mr Oldham thought that he was more likely to return to check when he was under stress, alone in the house or the office, or physically near to the object of his concern. He was less vulnerable if he was occupied with something else which held his interest, such as playing the piano, or if someone else assumed the responsibility for safety. Thus, he often persuaded his secretary to take charge of security and safety in the office and tried to get his wife to do the same at home.

Post-traumatic stress disorder (PTSD)

Although there has long been an awareness of neurotic disorders following psychological trauma, PTSD has only been recognized as a discrete anxiety disorder since 1980 when it was defined in DSM-III (American Psychiatric Association 1980). The characteristic features of the disorder are the development of recurrent and intrusive recollections and/or recurrent dreams of the event, with or without vivid flashbacks. There is also some emotional numbing and hyperalertness or sleep disturbance. Guilt, memory impairment, and avoidance of triggers for the memories are also characteristic.

PTSD is linked with a wide range of stressors: involvement in warfare (Freud *et al.* 1921) and more recently in Vietnam (Williams 1980; Atkinson *et al.* 1984); incarceration in prison camps (Kinzie *et al.* 1984); civil violence (Loughrey *et al.* 1988); natural disasters (Cowell McFarlane 1988); and rape (Rothbaum *et al.* 1990).

The therapist's role in treatment of PTSD is first, to help the survivor review memories of the trauma while expressing the appropriate affect. Then the client needs to desensitize to the traumatic memories and regain a sense of control.

A case of PTSD: Mr Thomas

Mr Thomas was 32 years old when he was involved, and injured, in a road traffic accident. Several months later, his physical condition was much improved, but he was still troubled by recurrent, involuntary memories of his accident, and by recurrent worries and guilt.

The memories were very vivid and triggered panic. They were set off by any reminder of the accident: traffic-lights changing, the noise of metal against metal, the smell of petrol, a newspaper report of a car accident. He avoided situations which would trigger his distress, he did not drive, and he certainly never went along the stretch of road where the accident happened. He would only travel by car if his wife drove, because he thought her a good driver, and would only use the new 'tank-like' family car. Sometimes memories came back as nightmares and, as a result, he was waking and agitated throughout the night, tired throughout the day. He was also troubled by a constant, nagging thought that, had his 4-year-old son been in the car with him, he would certainly have been killed. Now, Mr Thomas was reluctant to let his son travel, unless driven by his wife, and this was very restricting.

He was also plagued by feelings of guilt because a cyclist had been severely injured when his car was pushed sideways and he could not forgive himself for this. The thought that ran through his mind was 'I should have been more alert; I should have taken some action to save the cyclist: it is my fault that she will never walk again: people will hate me for this'. The image of the cyclist's body, crushed under the car, plagued him and featured vividly in his dreams.

Over the months, he had grown irritable and detached from his wife and family. He began to experience other recurring thoughts, which concerned his fitness to be a father and his self-worth: 'I could have killed my son because of my stupidity. I am a hopeless and dangerous father, a pathetic, stupid creature'. His mood had become depressed and it was for this reason that he sought help from his doctor.

'Executive stress' or 'burn out'

This is a term which has been coined to describe an extreme reaction to chronic stress. The term 'burn out' is not reserved for executives but was, in fact, first used to describe a syndrome common among caring professions such as teachers, doctors, clergy, and social workers (Freudenberger 1974). It is notable that these professions have higher than expected rates of suicide and alcohol or drug abuse (Maslach and Pines 1979).

The symptoms of 'executive stress' or 'burn out' are similar to the symptoms of the other stress disorders, the difference is that they tend to be ignored until the stress response is very marked. Most vulnerable are those who label the stress 'excitement', enjoying living on the cusp of the performance curve. Executive stress has been linked with personality type and physical illness. In the mid-sixties, Rosenman and co-workers identified a 'type A' personality which seemed to be more susceptible to coronary heart disease. The 'type A' person is competitive, high-achieving, impatient, and deeply involved in his or her work. The enjoyment of the job leads to their ignoring stress symptoms in the drive to achieve. Such relentless driving behaviour has also been linked with high blood pressure, raised cholesterol levels, and smoking—all of which impair health. Burn out also affects those with low job satisfaction. Perhaps a career plateau has been reached or a job lacks autonomy or is insecure. In this instance, an individual is likely to express job dissatisfaction and frustration.

A case of executive stress: Dr Evans

Dr Evans was a very successful, 35-year-old research officer, working for a multinational computer firm. Her job required her to travel a good deal in Britain and abroad.

She consulted her GP because she thought that she was, perhaps, going mad. She described a recent incident when she had to get to an important board meeting in order to report back on a conference which she had just attended in Geneva. Her flight from Geneva had been delayed by 10 hours and so she organized her presentation on the plane intending to go straight to the board meeting, rather than stopping off at her hotel first. She landed in London and planned to catch the train into town. There was a 15-minute wait and so she hailed a taxi, instead. In the taxi, she continued to work on her presentation, but was very aware of the time. Driving into London at this time meant that she would be caught in the morning rush hour: she reprimanded herself for not waiting for the train.

She never considered telephoning to let someone know that she had been delayed and it did not occur to her to devise ways of postponing her presentation. The work she had done for the meeting was good and she wanted to be seen presenting it. She felt excited by the thought of herself entering the meeting at 9.00 a.m., against all odds.

Then she began to feel too hot and had a ringing in her ears. She held on to the taxi seat because she was shaking and because she thought that she might fall. She could not catch her breath and the ringing in her ears became louder. She felt disorientated and helpless, all she could do was remain slumped in the seat hoping that this would pass. She also hoped that the taxi driver was unaware of her condition and concluded that she probably had not eaten enough on the plane.

Before they reached her destination, Dr Evans' symptoms had subsided but she felt shaken and annoyed that she had wasted so much time. She arrived at the meeting at 8.55 a.m., just in time to grab a coffee and a cigarette and to begin to feel elated by her achievement. Her presentation was well received and, by lunch-time, she was feeling very satisfied with herself. It was only now that she remembered to telephone her husband and children to let them know that she had landed safely.

Since then, she has experienced several more episodes of disorientation and ringing in her ears—none of which seemed to be related to hunger. Her conclusion was that she was going crazy and that this had to be put right.

Reactive anxiety

Symptoms of anxiety might be directly related to an identifiable incident, like the experience of redundancy threat, or health worries. In most cases the symptoms of anxiety diminish as the incident recedes into the past and only reassurance may be needed. Without coping skills, however, it is possible to develop a chronic and possibly disabling fear following a specific trauma.

No matter how appropriate an anxiety state seems, AMT employed soon after its onset can accelerate recovery and help prevent the development of a chronic problem. Intervention is known to be most effective near to a crisis, and health workers in close contact with people suffering from anxiety are in a special position to intervene.

Who is suitable?

There are certain features to look out for in the initial assessment which are likely to contra-indicate short-term AMT. Persons with a chronic history of anxiety and/or multiple phobias are often best referred to an agent who can offer long-term therapy. As a rule, the earlier the intervention, the more effective will be brief AMT.

If anxiety is clearly a secondary symptom of another problem, such as marital difficulties or interpersonal problems, then a different intervention might be appropriate, for example marriage guidance or psychotherapy. However, giving some additional help in coping with the anxiety symptoms can still be of benefit. A multiple-factor problem, where anxiety is only one aspect, might be most effectively dealt within long-term therapy. This is particularly the case for clients with personality disorders.

However, it is frequently impossible to establish the full situation in the first interview and complexities tend to emerge after a few sessions. For this reason, it is useful to arrange a contract of a limited number of appointments, after which progress can be reviewed and the method of approach reviewed according to the client's apparent needs.

As a general rule, it becomes evident within four to six sessions whether the client is suitable for this form of therapy.

2 *Control*

Introduction

Many people discover their own ways of coping with anxiety, such as regular breathing, relaxing, keeping active, or facing up to, rather than avoiding, their problems. In a 1990 community survey, Barker *et al.* discovered that the general population tends to resort to adaptive coping strategies using informal support networks. A tendency to avoid and a readiness to seek professional help was shown by those who reported more stress symptoms. Of those seeking help, some have never had the opportunity to develop useful coping skills or have tried these approaches without success. In cases where an anxious person is trying to use an innate coping strategy or is acting on advice, the technique may be abandoned. The most common reasons for giving up are:

(1) having too high expectations of the rate of efficacy, so that disappointment follows;

(2) having a poor understanding of the rationale of a coping technique and little faith in the exercise;

(3) using the approach incorrectly or incompletely.

In helping your client, it is important to teach the theory of the coping technique, the stages in the development of the practical skills and its proper mode of application. The key methods in psychological control involve:

- controlling bodily symptoms;
- controlling worrying thoughts;
- panic management.

Controlling bodily symptoms

In teaching the control of the somatic symptoms of anxiety, two techniques are useful: relaxation and controlled breathing.

Relaxation

Anxiety states are almost invariably associated with physical tension. It has been established that the autonomic effects accompanying muscular relaxation are directly antagonistic to those that characterize physical tension (Jacobsen 1938; Wolpe 1958). It is therefore reasonable to conclude that one can learn to control the somatic symptoms of anxiety by mastering relaxation. Few people know what to do when simply told to 'relax', and teaching them to do this entails careful tuition, allied to a training programme. The goal of therapy is to develop a skill which can be applied to the situation which triggers anxiety.

Forms of relaxation training vary. Included in the range of relaxation techniques are yoga, autogenics, meditation, and hypnotically induced relaxation. Jacobsen, in the 1930s, was the first to develop a systematic programme of progressive muscular relaxation (PMR) to help his patients respond to physical stress by relaxing rather than tensing their muscles. Jacobsen suggested that individual muscle groups should be focused upon in a systematic fashion. His instructions were to tense and then to relax a specific part of the body. When relaxation of one muscle group had been achieved, the next group would be attended to. In this way, the patient would work from the feet and calf muscles up through the body until all muscles were relaxed. In doing so, the patient could learn to distinguish between tension and relaxation, and to respond to tension by relaxing the muscle.

Although PMR is a lengthy exercise, it is often the necessary starting point in relaxation training. However, as the goal of this intervention is the development of a portable skill which can be used as the need arises and with reasonable speed, the person engaged in training is taught ways of shortening the exercises. Eventually relaxation is achieved within a few minutes, and the cue for relaxing is muscular tension.

Since the 1930s, relaxation training has been successfully used in the treatment of a wide range of anxiety-related problems, such as general anxiety, phobias, sexual difficulties, insomnia, backache, headache, and hypertension. Relaxation training helps the client to become more aware of the onset of tension and offers a means of controlling it, thereby increasing confidence. The combination of relaxation and e sure to a stressful situation has proven to be a very effective anxi management technique (Rachman 1966) particularly where the pre dominant symptoms of anxiety are physiological (Ost *et al.* 1991; 1992). There is also a correlation between physical relaxation and mental tranquility (Benson 1975; Peveler and Johnston 1986) which further aids the client in combating anxiety.

The skill of relaxation is readily learnt by most people and has high face validity; it is therefore a useful first step in AMT.

Controlled breathing

Respiratory control has recently become a popular anxiety management technique (Clark *et al.* 1985; Salkovskis *et al.* 1986). The approach assumes that hyperventilation, or overbreathing, is a common problem which aggravates anxiety, and that this state can be alleviated by teaching correct breathing.

The increase in respiration rate results in excessive elimination of carbon dioxide and consequent alkalosis. This in turn causes unpleasant bodily sensations, such as palpitations, paraesthesia, breathlessness, dizziness, sweating, muscle spasm, and chest pain. Although transitory shallow breathing is a normal response to stress, protracted overbreathing seems to be triggered by the catastrophic misinterpretation of the physical symptoms of hyperventilation (Clark 1987).

A cycle of apprehension and overbreathing is set up, with the symptoms of hyperventilation augmenting the original fear, which may culminate in a panic attack. Where overbreathing is a feature of the problem anxiety management involves educating the client about the causes and consequences of hyperventilation and then teaching a method of controlling respiration rate.

Controlling worrying thoughts

As explained in Chapter 1, anxiety may take the form of worrying thoughts, ruminations, images or fantasies which are difficult to dismiss. Although the worrying cognitions might be odd or extreme, they are not necessarily very bizarre or fantastic ideas, but rather what Meichenbaum (1985) describes as an 'internal dialogue of worrying perceptions', which predisposes a person to high levels of anxiety.

se, thought management can be learnt in two ying thoughts are identified and then they are ontrolled.

rying thoughts

e essential first step in thought management and is often very difficult for the client. Frequently, thoughts are half-formed ideas or pictures; they come and go quickly and may have become so automatic that they are very difficult to distinguish as the trigger for stress. Monitoring thoughts at times of stress facilitates the identification of worrying cognitions. Various methods of monitoring can be used and some will be discussed in detail in Chapter 6. The recording of worrying thoughts can, in itself, reduce the distress they cause. This is because people tend to become more detached and objective about worrying cognitions as they develop an increased awareness of stressful thought patterns or images.

Countering or controlling the thoughts

Once the anxiogenic thoughts have been identified, techniques to counter them can be explored. There are several cognitive approaches to anxiety management; some are relatively brief (see Butler 1985) while others require commitment to more long-term therapy (see Beck and Emery 1985). Two techniques which can be applied as part of a brief intervention programme are distraction and challenging thoughts.

Distraction

It is based on the assumption that someone can only fully attend to a single thought at a given time. In theory, a worrying idea can be replaced by a neutral or pleasant concept. This displaces the anxiety-provoking thought and prevents the build up of anxiety and the development of cycles of stress. With practice, clients can learn to use a distraction strategy in response to disturbing cognitions. The most commonly used strategies are physical activity, refocusing and formal mental activity.

Physical activity as a distraction technique requires one to keep occupied in stressful situations. For example, handing round drinks at an anxiety-provoking party or washing the car can provide a means of distraction from worrying thoughts.

Refocusing requires the client to concentrate hard on some aspect of the environment. For example, someone might try counting the number of items in a shopping trolley at the supermarket check-out, or reading in detail the notices in the dentist's surgery if these were situations of stress.

Mental activity simply means engaging in a formal mental task such as making a shopping list, reciting poetry, or carrying out a mental arithmetic task.

The effectiveness of a distraction strategy is often idiosyncratic and it is important for the client to experiment with several ideas and establish which is best and under what circumstances. As a general rule, the more anxious the client the less likely she or he is to be able to use the psychologically sophisticated techniques. So, at times of marked stress, a person might resort to physical distraction rather than mental exercises. Ideally, the client should have a repertoire of distraction techniques which accommodates a range of settings and varying degrees of anxiety. For example, a range of techniques for boardroom tension might incorporate: uncurling and recurling paper clips (physical activity); counting the number letters on the distributed minutes (refocusing); and mental arithmetic (mental activity). A range of distractors for stress on the train could involve: taking a walk down the corridor (physical activity); counting the number of houses passed by the train (refocusing); and imaging the life-styles and occupations of fellow passengers (mental activity). It should be noted that distraction can be misused in order to avoid confronting a difficult situation. If a socially anxious man is always involved in handing round drinks at parties, rather than mixing with people, he is unlikely to overcome his basic fear. It is important to note and discourage this type of avoidance by devising graded exposure to the aversive situation (Chapter 3).

Challenging thoughts

Is an effective technique for controlling worrying thoughts for those who find distraction ineffective or insufficient. While distraction, used properly, is an effective technique for controlling worrying thoughts, for some people the actual content of a worrying thought has to be attended to and challenged before it loses its anxiogenic properties.

Under most circumstances, we do not attend to our thoughts, so it is impossible re-evaluate anxiety-provoking thinking patterns. Once worrying thoughts have been identified, however, the client can begin to reappraise them realistically and thereby prevent the development of a

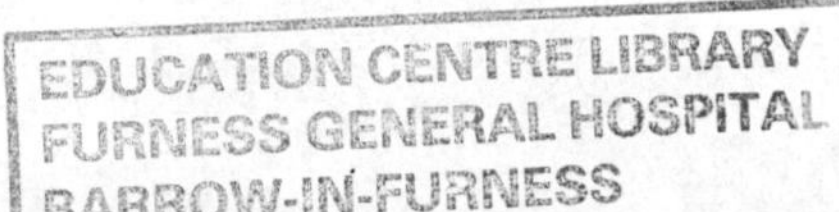

stress cycle. The thoughts, which are identified through diary keeping, are likely to contain what Beck and his co-workers (1979) call thinking errors. These are thoughts which are unrealistic, exaggerated, overly pessimistic, catastrophic, one-sided, categorical, and global. They therefore predispose a person to anxiety. Some examples of thinking errors are:

'Yesterday was terrible: *today is bound to be awful too*'.

'I feel faint, *therefore I am going to collapse and everyone will laugh at me*'.

'I stammered during my speech, *so I have ruined my daughter's wedding and she won't forgive me*'.

'My friend is late—*he's had an accident*'.

The aim of challenging is to reappraise worrying thoughts and reformulate them constructively. This technique has been shown to be an extremely effective anxiety management technique (Ellis 1962; Beck *et al.* 1979; Meichenbaum 1985). Challenging is not a matter of generating platitudes to gloss over the reality of a bad situation, but rather the realistic interpretation of events. The procedure involves analysing the thought and being rational about the worry. For example:

'Yesterday was terrible: *no, parts of it were good and although parts were uncomfortable, I coped*'.

'I feel faint: *I am probably anxious and I can control this*'.

'I stammered during my speech: *this is not the end of the world, it is common to get nervous when speaking in public*'.

'My friend is late:—*maybe he has been held up in the traffic, or has forgotten our date*'.

These kinds of statements need to be rehearsed while the individual is feeling calm, so that they can be readily employed at times of stress.

Images are challenged in a similar way, in that the worrying picture is modified by substitution of a non-alarming image. The anxiogenic image might present as a nightmare or a recurrent intrusive image or an image which is provoked by certain triggers. Whatever the presentation, once the client could describe the stressful content of the image, the therapist would help her or him to revise it, substituting masterful and positive images for the previously alarming ones.

Managing a panic attack

The principal aim of the techniques described so far is to prevent anxiety from developing. There are also techniques for controlling tension which has escalated into a panic attack. As stated earlier, hyperventilation has been associated with the onset of panic attacks. Slow breathing is incompatible with hyperventilation, and so training in slow, regular breathing has proved useful as a means of controlling the alarming physical symptoms of a panic attack (Clark *et al.* 1985). The other techniques which have been described are useful in panic management, but it is essential that they be well rehearsed before they are needed as it is difficult to apply the techniques during panic unless they have become almost automatic.

3 *Dealing with avoidance*

Introduction

Avoidance and loss of confidence are two of the consequences of anxiety. Since acute tension is so unpleasant, the natural reaction is to avoid whatever causes it. Avoidance can take the form of never confronting a situation, or only facing it while using a prop, such as drugs, alcohol, or a friend in order to minimize discomfort. This only serves to reduce one's confidence even further, and the problem worsens. A classic example of avoidance is an increasing reluctance to leave the home, which can develop into agoraphobia.

Even when a situation is not wholly avoided, the anxious person might face it for only a very short time, or might avoid the worst parts. For example, a man with a social phobia might attend a party but avoid conversation. By doing so, he does not learn his anxiety will subside if he perserveres in facing the fear, in fact, he reinforces 'I can't cope'.

The most effective means of overcoming both avoidance and loss of confidence has been shown to be exposure to the stressor which causes the anxiety. This almost always involves a systematic programme of planned practice or graded exposure.

Facing the fear: graded practice

Through graded exposure a person faces a feared situation in gradual stages. Practice is planned carefully so that the client experiences success with small tasks at first and builds on this success by going on to meet more difficult situations. These achievements also serve to enhance a sense of self-efficacy, perceived control, and personal responsibility, which in turn contribute to the re-establishment of self-confidence.

Graded exposure works by breaking the association between the feared situation and anxiety. It provides an opportunity to learn that the everyday situations or objects which cause anxiety are not really harmful. With carefully organized practice, a person can learn to face phobias and regain confidence.

In order to achieve this, each client needs a personal and structured programme of progressively more difficult tasks or activities which culminate in a specific goal. Exposure begins with the easiest task, which is planned so that it presents a challenge, but success is assured. Gradually, he or she progresses through a hierarchy of tasks until the goal is reached. Goals must be obtainable and objectives quantifiable. Emphasis is always on careful planning, as it is better to achieve something in a number of small successful steps than to risk failure by being over-ambitious.

Imagine that a man had an anxiety attack while signing a receipt in a busy shop and that his hand shook uncontrollably. He then became fearful of this happening again and avoided writing anything which might be witnessed. His goal in therapy, therefore, might be writing in public. This could be reduced to six steps:

(1) holding a pen without trembling, while alone;

(2) writing a short message, while alone;

(3) writing a short message, with one known person present;

(4) writing a short message, with a group of friends present;

(5) writing a short message, with a group of friends present but in a public place;

(6) writing a short message, without friends present and in a public place.

The first step, which must be achievable, is practised until the feelings of anxiety are controllable. Similarly, the next step is rehearsed until it presents little difficulty. This procedure continues until the goal is attained. Although it is necessary that goals be specific, there should be an element of flexibility so that adaptations can be made for unforseen problems. To be effective, the practice must be regular, and progress is likely to be enhanced if the client has basic coping skills. Exposure may take place in a variety of situations: in imagination, within the sessions, or outside the sessions.

In imagination

Imagery rehearsal, or facing a fear in imagination, has been successfully used to provide clients with an opportunity to develop coping skills (Wolpe 1958). This is usually carried out during a session, but can also be practised at home. As described earlier, the client and therapist develop a hierarchy of tasks, ranked in order of difficulty and culminating in a specified goal. The client relaxes and is then instructed to imagine the first stage in the hierarchy, while maintaining or returning to the relaxed state. When this can be achieved, the client progresses to the next task, and so on until the goal is reached. Meichenbaum (1971) established that the therapeutic value of imagery rehearsal is enhanced if the client visualizes becoming stressed and then imagines overcoming this.

The skills developed in imagery rehearsal are usually generalized to the real situation, so this method is particularly useful for helping people with fears which are not easily tackled *in vivo*. Examples of such phobias might be fear of flying, fear of snakes, or fear of thunder, where the phobic stimuli are too expensive, impractical, or unpredictable to tackle in sessions or as regular homework tasks. Imagery work is also a useful prelude to tackling a particularly aversive phobia. For example, Mrs Smith, described on page 22, was so fearful of wasps that she needed exposure in imagination to prepare her for the exposure *in vivo*.

Beck *et al.* (1985) outline the diversity of imagery work in anxiety management. Once the anxiogenic picture has been fully recognized, it can be modified through a range of techniques such as: 'turning off' alarming images by using forms of distraction—this is especially pertinent to PTSD; repeating the alarming image but systematically changing or 'decatastrophizing' the content so that it becomes less anxiety provoking; or 'time projecting' into the future in order to gain detachment from the image.

Another way to accomplish skills training away from the real situation is to role-play difficult situations with clients, while they use anxiety management techniques to cope with the stress that this evokes. Rehearsing public speaking or social interaction lends itself well to this method.

In the session

Some anxieties, such as fears of objects or small animals and some performance fears, can be dealt with during the therapy session. Again, a programme of practice is developed and supervised by the therapist during the session. A combination of exposure in the session and *in vivo* is often an effective way of tackling phobias. Someone who is fearful of eating in public might first practise in sessions and then move on to practising in real life situations.

Bandura (1970) proposed a further effective way in which the client and therapist could work together in the session, namely, modelling. This requires the therapist to carry out each step in the hierarchy in front of the client, who then copies the action. This might involve the therapist's handling an animal, writing while being observed, swallowing mouthfuls of food, or speaking on the telephone. Again, this is combined with anxiety management. A useful variation is modelling by using a video film which demonstrates coping with different stresses. This widens the number of fears which can be tackled in session work, as films can illustrate coping with public transport, shopping in a busy supermarket, or other stressful activities which could not normally be modelled in a session.

Outside the session

This is probably the most frequent place of practice and often the nature of the fear dictates that it be carried out *in situ*. Fear of travelling on trains or writing a cheque in the bank would be typical examples. The client is prepared in the sessions, and is helped to devise a programme of planned practice. The task is then carried out in the real situation in the form of graded homework assignments. He or she monitors progress and discusses it with the therapist at the next session.

These three approaches can, and sometimes should, be combined for optimum outcome, bearing in mind that the more similar the training session is to the actual situation, the greater the likelihood of success. Real-life exposures are more effective than exposure in imagination and carrying out homework in the real world is more effective than limiting exposure to the sessions.

Facing the fear: flooding

An alternative way of learning how to face a feared object or situation is by taking on the task at the top of the hierarchy immediately. This can be in imagination, known as implosion, or in reality when it is referred to as flooding.

In flooding, the individual is required to stay in an unpleasant situation. In theory, the anxiety eventually falls and he or she learns that nothing dreadful has happened as a consequence of remaining there. However, the experience is usually very stressful to the client and there is always a risk that he or she will not relax in the situation, or might retreat before the fear has subsided. If that should happen, then the client's anxiety is reinforced.

Flooding should not be undertaken without the client's consent and certainly only with persons who are well trained in relaxation techniques and who have been thoroughly prepared for a possibly violent reaction.

Facing the fear: problem solving

Sometimes a fear has to be faced at a predetermined time; weddings, examinations, or flights are not negotiable. On these occasions, there is often too little time to complete a programme of graded exposure.

At such time, problem solving is a useful means of enhancing your client's coping skills (Goldfried and Davidson 1976; D'Zurilla and Nezu 1982). Training in problem solving involves learning a sequence of steps in order to generate solutions to the problem. Anxiety is often reduced simply by having a set structure to follow. The steps in problem solving are:

1. Define the problem: ask what, when, who, where.
2. List solutions: as many as possible.
3. Rank solutions: in order or usefulness or ease.
4. Take the first solution.
5. Plan: decide what, when, who, where, how.
6. Implement the plan: do it.
7. Evaluate: did it work? If not, take the next solution on the list, and work down again from step 5.

The most important points to remember are: only a single and very specific problem should be taken on at any time. This might mean teasing out several problems and repeating the problem-solving exercise for each. Any solution can be generated in the process of brainstorming, no matter how bizarre—in fact these can often prove most useful; disappointments are to be expected and need not be disheartening as it is usually possible to learn from set-backs; perseverance should be encouraged.

Once a person has evolved a psychological conceptualization of her or his problem, and has attained skills in graded exposure and problem solving she or he can begin to build up confidence about facing difficult situations.

4 *Self-management and ending therapy*

Introduction

Throughout the programme, emphasis is always placed on the client's responsibility in taking control of the problem. The client is involved at all stages, from the assessment phase when self-monitoring of symptoms or thoughts is carried out, to the implementation of planned practice programmes, which are ultimately designed and executed by the client.

Once coping skills have been learned, clients can take full responsibility for using them. With practice, they become competent and confident in anxiety management, the skills become easier to use and are generalized to other situations.

The ability to cope can also be enhanced by changes in life-style, such as increasing social activity, and through changes in attitude—becoming more assertive, developing better sleep patterns, improving time management for example.

Withdrawal of medication

It is during this time that medication can be reduced or phased out completely because the client's confidence in coping with anxiety is increasing. This can be carried out with the support of a single health professional, or by joining a tranquillizer withdrawal support group, for example.

Relapse prevention

At some time, your client will experience successes which cannot be sustained. This might happen during the period of your involvement or after the course of AMT has finished. Everyone goes through bad patches, so it is advisable to prepare your client for an erratic course of progress. It is common for clients to hope for linear progress in therapy, but the most likely pattern of progress is a series of ups and downs and the client should be primed to expect the occasional set-back and to use it as a learning opportunity. If a person is not prepared for these, demoralization and rejection of anxiety management can result. It is possible, in the final sessions, to prepare your client for coping with set-backs in the absence of your direct support by helping her or him to anticipate difficulties and generate solutions to them. This is often referred to as blueprinting, and is most helpful if the difficulties and solutions are recorded for reference, rather than simply being committed to memory. In a crisis, memory is likely to be impaired, whereas a written list of coping strategies can be referred to at any time.

Therapy can be terminated when your client has a psychological model of coping with anxiety, can practise techniques with some success, can predict difficulties, and plan how to cope.

5 *Summary of Part I: Background Information*

Summary of Chapter 1: Anxiety

Anxiety is a normal reaction to stress which comprises behavioural, bodily, and mental components. Anxiety only becomes a problem when it is an unrealistic or unnecessarily persistent response. In some instances, the experience of anxiety can itself become a source of distress and the sufferer develops anxiety about anxiety.

The condition may manifest itself as free-floating anxiety, specific fears, panic attacks, post-traumatic stress, 'burn out', or it may be indicated by obsessional-compulsive behaviours. Each of these types of anxiety may be helped by using anxiety management training (AMT); however, the suitability of a person for therapy and the treatment approach to be adopted depends very much on the characteristics of that individual.

The decision to take on a client for AMT must follow a thorough investigation of all possible relevant information.

Summary of Chapter 2: Control

The three main methods of psychological control are:

(1) control of physical symptoms;

(2) control of worrying thoughts;

(3) control of panic.

These skills can be taught to, or enhanced in the client and then used to effect behavioural and/or emotional change. The choice of approach will depend on her or his needs and strengths, and the techniques may be used in combination.

Control of physical symptoms involves the client's learning sufficient muscular control to achieve a relaxed state which is incompatible with physical tension, and teaching a method of controlled breathing which is incompatible with hyperventilation. In thought management the client learns techniques to identify and combat distressing thoughts, ruminations, or fantasies. Panic management involves preparing the client to control tensions which have escalated into a panic attack.

Summary of Chapter 3: Dealing with avoidance

Carefully planned exposure to the feared object or situation breaks its association with anxiety. Exposure provides the client with an opportunity to learn that a feared situation holds no real personal harm. Repeated exposure strengthens this belief, and builds up lost confidence.

The key factors when using graded exposure are:

(1) individual planning;

(2) progress through graded, achievable steps: no risk taking;

(3) building on success;

(4) repeated practice;

This can take place:

(1) in imagination;

(2) in the session—including modelling;

(3) in real life.

Summary of Chapter 4: Self-management and ending therapy

In summary, the aim of anxiety management is to prepare the client to cope with anxiety independently. This means that the client must achieve the following:

(1) an understanding of the concept of normal and abnormal anxiety;

(2) the ability to apply anxiety management skills in the context of need;

(3) the capacity to anticipate and manage new problems;

(4) the ability to modify her/his outlook and life-style in order to minimize unnecessary stress;

(5) the confidence to do all this alone.

The goal of the therapist is to help the client reach this stage.

PART II

Preparatory notes for the therapist

6 *Anxiety*

The assessment

Before starting an anxiety management programme, it is important to consider which coping methods are suitable for your client. There is no one-to-one relationship between the use of any single form of coping and good results. Factors associated with success under one set of circumstances might not be successful at another time. In order to establish the particular training needs of a client, the therapist must gather sufficient data about the problem to arrive at a formulation and sufficient information about the person to decide on the optimum approach for her or him. The necessary information is compiled through interview, self-monitoring tasks, and observation.

Most people feel more able to disclose details of a problem to a warm, empathic, and non-judgemental assessor who communicates concern and is encouraging if they find discussion difficult. It is important not only to listen carefully, but also to check your understanding of the details by summarizing and reflecting back the client's statements. It is worth remembering the point made by Miechenbaum (1985), that psychological assessment is not a cross-examination, but an 'organized, systematic attempt to better understand the client's stress and coping experiences'.

Collecting information in the assessment

Anxiety rarely falls into neat categories. Broadly speaking, the aim of the therapist in the assessment of anxiety is to collect sufficient information to develop a formulation of a particular individual's problem. Devising a psychological treatment plan depends less on the diagnosis than on the practical assessment of the way anxiety affects someone's life, and on that person's potential to change. Therapy focuses on specific difficulties and not general problems.

Once you have decided that your client has an anxiety-related problem, it is necessary to collect sufficient information to understand the problem fully. If you are a GP, it is most likely that your client will present the problem in a standard consultation session and so you might not be able to carry out the assessment immediately. It is probably best to make a return appointment for a longer session when you can collect the information that you need to make a formulation of the problem and develop a treatment plan. Other professionals may have more flexible schedules and thus be able to carry out the assessment when the problem is presented.

Whatever the circumstances of the assessment period, do not be afraid of taking time over the procedure—this initial data collection is extremely important and should not be superficial. Basing your treatment plans on insufficient information could result in excessive revisions of your approach, which is time-consuming and demoralizing for both the client and therapist. At worst, you could develop the wrong treatment approach and find yourself unable to help your client.

Bear in mind that your client should have a clear idea of the function of the assessment session. An understanding of the function and format of the session will reduce anxiety, prepare the client for the collaborative relationship necessary for AMT, and begin the process of education. If you need to make a return appointment, your client can carry out a self-monitoring task in the intervening time.

An assessment should cover the following points.

1. The presenting problem

Find out more about the client's view of the problem and the reasons for seeking help. You could ask your client to describe a recent experience so that you get a clearer understanding of what the anxiety comprizes in terms of the behavioural, somatic, and cognitive elements. Also, elicit details of the duration of the problem or an episode, the frequency of the anxiety attacks, and the severity of these experiences. Find out what events or situations trigger, exacerbate, or ameliorate the problem condition.

2. The history of the problem

It is important to know what predisposes particular individuals to their problems, in other words, what makes a certain person vulnerable. Factors to note may be personal, such as character traits or early experiences, or family factors such as personality traits of family members or the family dynamics.

When compiling a brief history, establish the circumstances contributing to the development of the problem and the onset factors. What was happening in your client's life around the time the problem began? Then enquire about the course of the difficulty: has this been chronic or intermittent, for example?

3. Current coping methods

Discover the person's own coping methods, and classify them according to their long-term usefulness. You can do this by asking the client to recall what she or he does in response to the problem and supplement the information through diary keeping. Once you are both aware of the client's coping methods, you can decide which are appropriate or adaptive coping methods (e.g. relaxation) as you may be able to help the person to use these more efficiently. Also establish which coping methods are harmful or maladaptive (e.g. alcohol use) as these need to be phased out and replaced by appropriate or adaptive coping methods. It can be demoralizing for a client to learn that her or his methods of coping are 'maladaptive' as this is often construed as a failing. It can be more helpful to refer to coping strategies as those which are effective in the short-term and those which have long-term benefits. It is also important not to give the impression that maladaptive coping strategies will be banned immediately. This can be alarming for a client who cannot envisage coping without the help of reassurance or a drink etc., and is likely to affect level of motivation.

4. Relevant investigations

Your client may have been subject to previous psychological investigation. This could have been neuropsychological, behavioural, or intellectual assessment, or an assessment of affect. Findings from such investigations will contribute to your understanding of the particular strengths, needs, and possible limitations of your client. For example, someone with mild or moderate depression could be intellectually and physically retarded, or a person with learning difficulties might have difficulty keeping diaries.

Similarly, he or she might have had certain medical investigations. The results of these could help you to rule out an organic aetiology, while learning more about the person's physical state may give insight into limitations of therapy. For example, someone with gastro-oesophageal reflux might find it difficult to lie down for relaxation training.

5. Previous treatment

It is possible that your client has had previous psychological intervention, the outcome of which will further help you to formulate that person's problem. You might also gain some indication of the approaches which have helped in the past, and which you could incorporate in your treatment. For example, you might discover that someone has responded to progressive muscular relaxation training and you might then usefully build on this. Other treatments to note might include pharmacological or homeopathic therapies or help from practitioners such as an acupuncturist or chiropractor.

6. Current involvement of other agencies

It is essential to note what other medical, paramedical, and non-medical agencies are involved in the management of your client's anxiety. In some instances this may be complementary involvement, while the concurrent work of others might confuse you therapy. For example, the involvement of a social worker who can sort out your client's chronic housing problem is likely to enhance your client's recovery, while the ongoing involvement of another personal therapist might well make it very difficult for you to evaluate your progress with AMT; another therapist might even be using an intervention which conflicts with your approach.

7. Current medication

If you are the client's GP, you will probably be familiar with her or his medication and the possible effects it has on that person's anxiety state. If there are side-effects which could be misinterpreted for anxiety symptoms, it is important that your client knows this. As the therapist, you should be aware of the physical and cognitive consequences of any drug being taken by your client.

Also under this category, it is as well to note the use of other substances which may enhance the somatic features of anxiety. These will include caffeine, alcohol, cigarettes, or substances which your client is using in self-medication.

8. Your client's expectations of treatment and motivation to change

It is important to know what your client expects of treatment, such as duration, degree of active involvement, or degree of unpleasantness, so that you can identify any incorrect expectations. It is also necessary to know what your client believes would help as there may be misconceptions about treatment which should be clarified. For example, your client might believe that drugs or indefinite friendly chatting is the answer to the problem, while the therapist will be offering a quite different approach. Find out, also, what the client's hopes are regarding coping with the anxiety. Someone may expect to be completely anxiety-free or think that managing anxiety is an effortless task. Use this opportunity to make clear the realities of anxiety management and try to assess how motivated your client is to follow such a procedure.

9. Personal targets of change

The therapist needs to know what the client hopes to achieve in treatment. The therapist can ask, 'What do you expect to be able to do by the end of therapy?' The aim of this question is to elicit specific and realistic goals of therapy. Unrealistic expectations of treatment can be corrected at this early stage and vague goals can be made more definite.

10. Other relevant details

If you are not already familiar with your client's current psychosocial state, it is worthwhile making a note of current mood, current social, family, and marital situation (including available social support) and current employment status. Such factors can limit or enhance your AMT work, and it is important for you to be aware of them. This will be discussed more fully with respect to the evaluation of resources.

Collecting information: assessment of the client's strengths and needs

You will have to address the questions: 'What assets can we build on in therapy?', and 'What deficits need to be redressed and what behaviours should be discouraged?'. This involves reviewing personal assets and deficits while considering what external influences exist, which might contribute to or hinder the progress of your client.

The information you need to make judgements about your client's strengths and needs will have been collected during the assessment of the problem anxiety. When you have this information, there are four particular factors to be considered.

The first of these is the outcome goal which might well differ in the short term in comparison with the long term. For example, a woman may benefit from distraction training to help her get through an isolated difficult social situation, but would need to learn thought challenging to cope with a chronic worry that people were laughing at her.

Secondly, the timing of the intervention must be taken into account. If a person has to cope with a wedding next week, then a problem-solving approach would be more useful than a graded exposure plan, which might not be completed before the wedding day.

Thirdly, the context of coping should be considered. In some situations, it is possible to combat hyperventilation by breathing into a paper bag but, during a dinner party, controlled breathing is generally more acceptable.

Fourthly, each person's resources must be evaluated. Resources can be personal or external. When considering personal resources, remember that your clients are likely to have developed their own ways of coping with their anxiety. It is necessary to establish which of these methods are sound, adaptive, coping techniques and which are potentially harmful to them, or maladaptive. Examples of adaptive coping methods include rational thinking, adopting a problem-solving approach, or taking a relaxed attitude to minor stress. Some examples of maladaptive coping strategies are avoidance, substance abuse, and excessive dependency on others. A treatment programme should be designed to build on existing adaptive methods and encourage the development of new ones, while discouraging over-dependence on maladaptive techniques.

Other factors, such as character traits, will have an impact on treatment. Personal strengths such as high motivation, planning skills, or an ability to learn quickly can be exploited in AMT; however, you may also have to accommodate personal needs, for example the need for a simply presented programme or for a great deal of encouragement.

External resources concern factors which are external to the individual but which can be incorporated into the programme in order to maximize its efficiency. These could be assets such as supportive friends or family who are willing to be involved in the treatment, or more practical resources such as the use of a car or the ability to pay for repeated trips on public transport in order to carry out exposure tasks. When considering assets, it is just as important to note constraints such as low income or the lack of a babysitter, which could limit the scope of AMT.

As it is difficult to get more than just a feel for a problem in a single session, you might find that you need to arrange a further meeting for assessment. The amount of detail to be collected will vary for each client. Certain areas of the assessment can be abridged depending on the individual and the problem.

Although not compulsory, it is worthwhile to ask the client to complete some form of anxiety checklist. Two of the most commonly used questionnaires which you might find useful were developed by Speilberger and co-workers (1983) and Beck *et al.* (1986). Ratings from the checklists give an indication of the current state of anxiety and provide a baseline against which to compare progress. If used, a checklist should be administered regularly, preferably at each meeting.

Education

Assessment sessions present an opportunity to begin educating your client about the psychological interpretation of anxiety, the development of problem anxiety, and its management through self-help. The assessor should be familiar with the *client information sheet* (Client Information Sheet 1 on pages 00 and 000) which describes the psychological model of anxiety. If time permits, it is useful to go through this sheet in the session to check on the client's understanding of the model. Alternatively, the information can be read at home and if there are any points of confusion, they can be clarified at the next meeting. The appropriate information is given in Client Information Sheet 1.

Developing a formulation

You can use the information collected in the assessment sessions to make a formulation of the problem and a management plan for the future. Remember that a formulation is a definition of the client's problem within her or his own context. The construction of a formulation involves good history taking and a sound understanding of the client. Once the assessment has been made, the formulation which follows should contain the salient aetiological factors, as well as the strengths and needs of this person. The formulation is used to generate hypotheses about the maintenance of the problem. This then leads to a plan of treatment which is considered in terms both of the ideal and then what is possible given the constraints acting upon and the facilities available to this individual.

The formulation should be prepared with a view to presenting it to the client. The formulation is useful in making seemingly chaotic and unpredictable events understandable and predictable for the client (and the therapist!). By discussing it you can be certain that you have a shared rationale for the treatment plan. You should also remember that a formulation is dynamic: it is a working hypothesis which can be altered at any stage, with an appropriate revision of the management plan. Figure 6.1 shows a formulation in its simplest format.

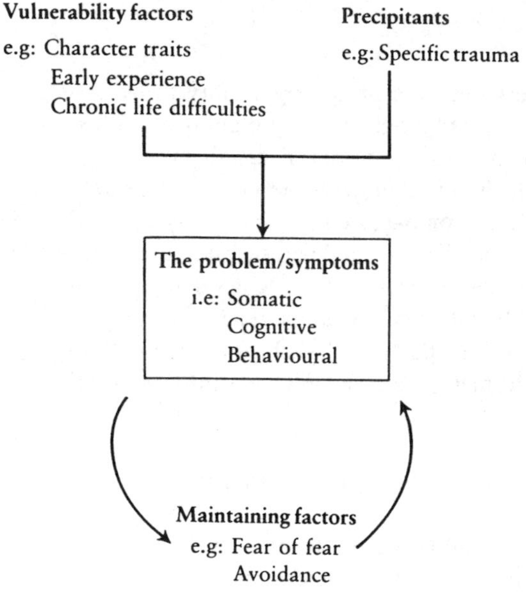

This will lead on to your:
Management plan
e.g: Relaxation
Graded exposure

Which is influenced by:
Modifying factors
e.g: Yoga skills
Supportive partner
Low income

Fig. 6.1 How to make a formulation

You may, for example, encounter a youth complaining of 'a fear of dogs' and your diagnosis of the problem might be one of simple phobia. Following your assessment of his phobia, you might have gathered the following information.

The presenting problem

Somatic symptoms—difficulty breathing, tingling in hands and legs, dizziness and faintness, sweating, muscle tremor.

Cognitive symptoms—thoughts that dogs will always bite; fears of madness; fear of passing out.

Behavioural symptoms—fleeing from the area and subsequent avoidance.

Symptoms are more intense when the client is stressed or tired and when he anticipates being near to a dog.

History of problem

The client reported being a 'nervous' child who was badly bitten by a dog when 4 years old; his mother was disturbed by this and displayed symptoms of panic when near dogs.

Current coping methods

Valium, alcohol, avoidance (maladaptive); tries to tell himself to be rational (adaptive).

Other treatment

He has taken Valium in the past.

Mood

Mild depression, secondary to anxiety.

Goals

To walk to the local pub alone without feeling anxious; to go jogging in the park where dogs are exercised.

Other information

Only child; protective mother; PE student at local college; no other problems; now seeks help because he has a girl-friend and wishes to be less socially restricted with her.

Resources
Well motivated; has supportive girl-friend who will be prepared to help with homework tasks.

You could now develop a preliminary formulation. It seems probable that this man has a predisposition towards anxiety and developed an intense and irrational fear of dogs following a traumatic personal experience. This was likely to have been intensified by his mother's anxious response. Thus, he learnt to fear dogs together with a panic response to them. His fear aroused somatic symptoms which eventually developed into panic attacks. These in themselves became aversive and he also grew fearful of panic attacks. His predominant coping response was avoidance and therefore he never learned that it might be safe to walk in the open, or that panic attacks can be controlled. He is now most vulnerable to anxiety symptoms when under stress or when tired.

At this stage, you could present your interpretation, but you might now realize that more information is needed about your client's cognitive coping strategies as you are unsure whether or not they are helpful. You could, therefore, present the formulation to check out its accuracy and acceptability, and then collect more information to update it. This could be compiled through interview or by suggesting that your client keep a thought diary.

Once you are agreed on the accuracy of the formulation, you are in a position to consider the appropriate intervention and necessary teaching which will enable you to help your client attain the specified goals. Remember to consider your client's special needs or limitations. In this example, it would be necessary to consider the impact of mood and living with an overprotective, dog-phobic mother. It would also be important to examine how the physical exertion demanded by a PE course might tire the man and contribute to his vulnerability to anxiety. You should determine how great is his dependency on Valium and alcohol as you need to know if you will have to help him cope with withdrawal symptoms too. There are also his particular assets to consider. He probably has a good understanding of the mechanism of the body, which could be useful when teaching control of somatic symptoms, and he seems to have found some benefit from using his own cognitive techniques which could be developed further. As his girl-friend is prepared to be involved, she could take part in a graded exposure programme.

The therapist's main focus is usually those factors which perpetuate the problem, as the maintaining factors are prominent in determining the type of intervention. However, when presenting the formulation, it is worth bearing in mind that the client is often more interested in the history of the problem the therapist needs to bear this in mind, particularly at the beginning of therapy when the validity of intervention and a working alliance are being established.

Goal setting in the assessment session

From the very beginning, the client should be encouraged to be specific and realistic when defining goals or targets of change. It is necessary to identify detailed goals for each problem, rather than devising vague targets such as: 'Overcoming my agoraphobia' or even 'Going shopping again'. A more useful target is: 'Going into the local supermarket, alone, on a weekday afternoon'. When goals are specific, the client and therapist have a shared and unambiguous aim in therapy. They can recognize quite clearly when the target has been reached and can then evaluate progress. In addition, by discussing goals the therapist can ensure that the client has a reasonable idea of what can be achieved through anxiety management.

Essential components of any AMT programme

Diary keeping

A major feature of AMT is therapist–client collaboration. Diary keeping, set as homework from the first session, encourages this working alliance and early diaries provide a baseline from which progress can be monitored. Such self-monitoring involves the client keeping systematic records of anxiety. This can range from marking stress levels on a simple visual analogue scale to filling in very detailed and specific records of the experience of anxiety. The latter are most useful in the early stages of therapy, as they yield much information. The incorporation of recordings of the events preceding an anxiety attack and the consequences of that anxiety, give further information which can help to clarify the problem for both the therapist and client. A typical anxiety diary is shown in Fig. 6.2. Whatever the type of scale used, instructions for its completion must be unambiguous and as simple as possible. It is wise to check that your client understands how to complete a recording schedule by working through an example in the session.

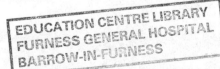

Anxiety record

Note down all the occasions when you experienced anxiety. Note them immediately after they happen or, if this is not possible, at the end of the day. *Do not leave it more than a day.* Rate your anxiety on each occasion on the following scale

0	1	2	3	4	5	6	7	8	9	10
No anxiety, calm					Moderate anxiety					Absolute panic, worst possible

Record what brought on the anxiety (in terms of thoughts or fantasies, or specific events or situations) and what you did in response. Then re-rate your level of anxiety.

Date/ Time	Describe the occasion when you experienced the anxiety	Rating (0–10)	What brought about the anxiety – thoughts, events	What did you do	Rating now (0–10)
DIARY 1			Please bring this to your next appointment		

Fig. 6.2 An anxiety diary

The recorded information might concern general feelings of anxiety, anxiety-provoking thoughts, or somatic symptoms (Diaries 1, 2, and 3 in Appendix 7). The diary you choose will depend on the particular problem under investigation: do you want to know more about the general level of anxiety or a specific aspect, such as thoughts or neck pain?

When people record events, the frequency of those events often changes. The rate of nail biting in a nervous student might decrease because a previously automatic response to stress is interrupted by the process of recording the behaviour. In contrast, the rate of food consumption in a person who binges in response to stress might increase because that person becomes preoccupied with food during the period she carries around an eating diary. None the less, diary keeping is worthwhile because it is the source of much information, and behaviour change is often in the therapeutic direction (Kazdin 1974).

Compliance with self-monitoring tasks gives an indication of a person's limitations or motivation. Difficulties and resistance to treatment at this stage should be explored, as you may need to reappraise your approach. An anxiety record which is not completed is perhaps too detailed and confusing for someone who is unfamiliar with diary keeping and a simpler one is needed. Alternatively, the A4-size diary might be too indiscreet for some clients who would prefer to use an index-card-size record. There are those who do not complete records because they have a fear of failing or a fear of being judged on the content of the diary. In these instances, a simple record of the number of thoughts, rather than the details of the cognitions, can be kept until the client feels more confident about disclosing.

Organization of appointments

The organization of appointments requires some long-term planning. Each client will require his or her own regimen; some may need close supervision, while others will be more independent. As a general guideline, sessions are usually weekly and need to be of sufficient length to review the experiences of the previous week and to plan the next stage.

It is important to give an idea of the overall structure of the programme. For example, indicate how many sessions there will be before a review, how frequent these will be, and how long a session will last. Uncertainty is anxiety provoking, especially for an already anxious client. To promote compliance, always set a date for the next appointment.

Setting contracts

It can be helpful to contract your client for a definite period of AMT, after which progress can be reviewed. The initial contract can cover any set period during which time the therapist can establish the appropriateness of treatment, discover the client's level of motivation, and prepare the client for a possible change in treatment plan in the future.

It is usual to offer a set number of sessions after which progress will be reviewed. In the review session a decision can be made to continue or to terminate therapy. Sometimes it is necessary only to offer a few appointments, for example, one or two 'booster' sessions subsequent to previous treatment, or a limited number of meetings, if you are aware that client is in danger of becoming overdependent.

Although members of a primary care team are likely to see practice patients for a number of different reasons, it can be made clear in setting the contract, whether verbal or written, that sessions set aside for AMT are only for this purpose and are not general consultation sessions. Emphasize that, for the period of therapy, the two are distinct.

Assessment and formulation: case examples

A case of generalized anxiety: Mrs Green

Mrs Green had given her GP a brief description of the physical symptoms of her anxiety, the thoughts which ran through her mind, and the behaviour which she displayed when experiencing an anxiety attack. At the initial consultation session, the GP had also learnt that Mrs Green was smoking, using tranquillizers, and avoiding certain situations in order to combat her anxiety.

Collecting the relevant information

Prior to attempting to make a formulation, Mrs Green's GP arranged to see her for a history-taking session. She discovered that Mrs Green had been divorced for 15 years and had recently moved to the village. Her two children did not live close by, but kept in touch by telephone. She was the youngest of three academically gifted children. Her father died when she was in her early teens and her brother and sister had left home to attend university. At this time, her mother became very depressed and would take to her bed for several days at a time. The mother grew increasingly distressed and began to have inexplicable bouts of choking, which frightened Mrs Green because she believed her mother was about to suffocate. The mother also developed a fear of going outside, and was virtually housebound until her death. Mrs Green found herself in the role of carer to a very demanding mother, and she gave up her plans to go to university.

In her early twenties, Mrs Green married because she was pregnant and 'in order to escape from mother'. The relationship was not a happy one because Mr Green was a rather cold authority figure and gave his wife little emotional support. She was filled with guilt for abandoning her mother and for being pregnant. When she miscarried on the way to the maternity unit, she had her first panic attack. From this time onward, she describes herself as a very nervous person, with her anxiety becoming most severe and chronic during stressful periods in her life. The most notable were during her first pregnancy and throughout the period of her divorce. On each occasion, the very severe level of anxiety had remitted within a few weeks; however, this last episode had continued for almost 2 years.

Approximately 2 years ago, she experienced several stressful events. Her son married and moved away from home, at which point Mrs Green decided to buy a smaller house in the village where she had been a child, and where she had lived when she had first married. Although she had grown up in this village, she had lived elsewhere for 25 years and no longer felt part of the community. On the positive side, her daughter had given birth to Mrs Green's first grandchild, but the pregnancy had been complicated and Mrs Green had been stressed by the fact that she could not be near her daughter who lived in Scotland. She had become involved with the church community and derived some comfort and company from this. However, as her levels of anxiety had increased she had found herself less able to attend services and meetings, and was becoming more socially isolated. At the time of the interview, she felt that she had only a single friend and confidant in the village.

In order to find out more specific details of her problem, the GP had suggested that Mrs Green should keep a diary for a week and then bring it along to the history-taking session. Mrs Green had recorded the events which preceded an increase in her levels of tension; details of the actual experience in terms of physical and psychological symptoms; and what she did in response to the tension. From the diary, they both discovered that her anxiety fluctuated markedly over each day. This had surprised Mrs Green because she had been convinced that her levels of tension were constantly elevated. It appeared, from the diary, that her anxiety was most pronounced in anticipation of stresses. For example, her anxiety increased before going out, before meals, or prior to dealing with any problems. She was most relaxed when engaged in a pleasurable activity such as reading the Bible.

Formulating Mrs Green's problem

The GP was now able to offer her preliminary thoughts on the development and maintenance of the problem. She presented the following explanation.

Vulnerability factors Mrs Green had grown up with an anxious mother who both created anxiety in the family and modelled maladaptive coping. Mrs Green had expected to respond to stress in the same way. The chronic stress of caring for her mother, the anger and frustration at not being free to go to university, and the feelings of guilt about her pregnancy and leaving her mother combined to make her vulnerable to an anxiety-related problem. In addition, marital stress and lack of emotional support at a particularly difficult time in her life further increased the likelihood of such a problem emerging.

Precipitants In a state of chronic stress, the emotional and physical shock of the miscarriage precipitated her first panic attack, and set up a 'fear of fear' in Mrs Green. Since the first attack, major stresses such as pregnancy and divorce have triggered periods of anxiety. Recently, the strain of her son's leaving home and her house move, coupled with worry about her daughter and her own loneliness, were sufficient to trigger the generalized anxiety disorder.

Maintaining factors It seemed that the physical symptoms of anxiety, which were uncontrollable and frightening, were exacerbated by her worrying thought which included the fear of fear. In addition, her decreased self-confidence which had developed through avoidance made it even more difficult for Mrs Green to face her fear. Poor coping techniques (smoking, tranquillizers, and avoidance) handicapped Mrs Green in establishing adaptive self-help skills, and her social isolation, which was the result of her increasing avoidance, further undermined her ability to tackle her fear.

A case of simple phobia: Mrs Smith

The health visitor who had witnessed Mrs Smith's anxiety attack realized that it was important to present a preliminary formulation to her during this visit. The health visitor's expectation was that the formulation would explain the problem in psychosocial terms and reassure her client that she was not losing her mind.

Collecting the relevant information

By spending an extra half-hour with Mrs Smith, the health visitor was able to gather enough information to make a formulation of the problem. Mrs Smith described herself as having been an anxious child, who never felt loved by her cold and rejecting mother. She recalled that she and her two older sisters were fiercely reprimanded if they tried to cuddle their mother, and any show of affection was not reciprocated by her. Mrs Smith had never felt comfortable with any physical show of affection, especially hugging, although she made a tremendous effort to kiss and cuddle her own children so that they would not feel as rejected as she had. None the less, her automatic response was to recoil from being touched.

Along with her siblings, she had been afraid of insects as a child, but, unlike them, she had never outgrown her fears. She could remember that she once ran to her mother in distress because a wasp had brushed her skin, only to be shouted at and forced back into the garden. She continued to be fearful of wasps, and, from this time, began to develop an increasingly efficient system of avoidance.

The fear of wasps reached the level of severity seen by the health visitor during her third pregnancy. At this time, she was raising two toddlers while her husband was working abroad for a month. She was missing him, especially as they lived far from either of their families or her old circle of friends. She had felt very tired and nauseous in the early stages of this pregnancy. On a particularly sunny day, when she knew that there would be wasps outside, she stepped into the garden, to call to her children. She was suddenly overwhelmed by feelings or sickness. She retreated to the kitchen feeling very shaky and with no one to comfort her. From then on, going into the garden (which was already associated with wasps) triggered feelings of nausea.

Formulating Mrs Smith's problem

At the end of her visit, the health visitor was able to suggest the following explanation for Mrs Smith's problem, stressing that anyone who had experienced such events might well develop emotional problems.

Vulnerability factors Mrs Smith was a rather insecure child who was prone to worrying—this was the probable result of her being so frequently and violently rejected by her mother. The physical rebuffs she received helped her to develop an aversion to being touched. Like most children, she had a fear of wasps, which is very possibly innate—unlike many children, however, she did not lose this fear. This was partly because she was prone to worrying and, because of her experience, being touched by a wasp was linked with a scolding and rejection from her mother.

Precipitants When Mrs Smith walked into her garden, she was already anticipating seeing a wasp, and thus her anxiety was raised. She was also very vulnerable to feelings of nausea. This was during a time in her life when she was experiencing the psychological stress of raising two children without any support, and the physical stress of pregnancy. This combination of factors would be sufficient to trigger the anxiety attack which led to her developing an association between wasps and the garden and alarming symptoms of fear.

Maintaining factors The phobia seemed to be perpetuated by several factors. First, by the physical symptoms of anxiety which she could not control and which were exacerbated by her belief that she was going mad. Secondly, by the vivid mental picture she had of a wasp crawling on her, which was elicited by any thought of wasps, and which was anxiety provoking because of her aversion to being touched. Finally, by her avoidance of wasps, which minimized her opportunity to learn that she could cope with them.

Mrs Smith was fascinated by the formulation. She had never considered her problem in this way, and exclaimed, 'It makes sense, doesn't it? I'm not going mad'. She easily understood the structure of the formulation and was able to add a further trigger factor: she and her husband had argued before he left the country and this had been on her mind, thus rendering her even more vulnerable to anxiety.

A case of panic attack: Mr Peters

Mr Peters had lived in the same village nearly all his life and was well known by his GP. Therefore, she needed only spend a short session with him to collect sufficient information to formulate his problem.

Collecting the information

Using what she knew of him and details he gave her in the session, the GP was able to compile a history. Mr Peters was the only child of a farming couple. He seemed to have had a normal, happy childhood until he was 15 years old. At that time, he was studying at home for his `O' levels, when he heard a noise in the kitchen. He ran in to find his 58-year old father lying dead on the floor. The family had always presumed that Mr Peters senior was quite healthy, but he had suffered a cerebrovascular accident. Somehow, the teenage Mr Peters immediately took on the role of head of the household, supported his mother, and managed to take his school exams and achieve good grades. From his description it seemed that he had never really grieved for his father and had coped by shutting the incident out of his mind.

Mr Peters did well at university and was successful in his business career which involved travelling abroad and driving a great deal. He engaged in a lot of sport, and, unlike his father, he never smoked and he watched his diet assiduously. In his late twenties he married and had two children. Within a few years, his relationship with his wife had deteriorated, but they stayed together, agreeing that this was probably best for the children. By the time of their divorce, the relationship was very acrimonious and stressful. The divorce was precipitated by Mr Peter's decision to leave his first wife in order to live with his current spouse. When asked how he now felt about his first marriage, he said that he never looked back or dwelt on the past; to him the matter was closed. During this time of transition, he suffered from glandular fever and was forced to take 2 months sick leave. Soon after his recovery, Mr Peters experienced his first panic attack.

It was his first day back at work and he had begun the long drive home after an unsuccessful business deal in the city. His muscles ached, his neck was stiff, he began to gasp for breath, and the sensations grew progressively worse. That night, at home, he felt short of breath and continued to feel unwell for about 48 hours. He was extremely alarmed by this and dared not go out for his usual evening jog. A few days later he experience similar, but more severe sensations when returning home from Wales. On this occasion, he waited in a lay-by for 20 or 30 minutes until the sensations passed, after which time he felt exhausted and was convinced that he had experienced some form of heart attack. He grew more fearful of being away from home, yet forced himself to continue travelling long distances by car. He had several more similar attacks in the car before consulting his GP.

Formulating Mr Peter's problem

Given this information, his GP was able to compile a formulation of the problem and present it to Mr Peters.

Vulnerability factors Mr Peters had repressed a great deal of emotional trauma as a teenager, namely, his feelings about his father's death, caring for his widowed mother, and his exam stress. It seemed that his way of tackling emotional problems was to deny them, thus causing a build-up of tension. Following his father's sudden death, he developed fears about his own health which he kept under control by making a conscious effort to watch his diet and to exercise. In his thirties, Mr Peters had experienced chronic marital stress, which would further contribute to his vulnerability to developing a stress-related problem.

Precipitants Around the time of his first panic attack, there were several discrete events which could have acted as triggers. He was going through an unpleasant divorce, he suffered a debilitating illness, and on the day of the panic attack, he had experienced a particularly strenuous and disappointing return to work.

Maintaining factors The problem did not remit after this first attack for several reasons. Mr Peters developed a fear of physical symptoms which he could not control and which, in turn, triggered the anxiety symptoms. There was also, the GP thought, a good chance that he was hyperventilating in response to stress. In addition, his strong belief that he was likely to have a heart attack and die suddenly would maintain his anxiety levels, as would his tendency towards catastrophic thinking. Finally, he subjected himself to unhelpful exposure. He forced himself to take excessively long journeys and thus set himself up to panic, which demoralized him further and strengthened his belief that something terrible would happen to him.

The first step in the management of Mr Peter's problem was education. Using the formulation, his GP discussed the psychogenic origin of panic attacks in general, and then specifically in his case. Mr Peters accepted this model, especially the idea of his problem being maintained through vicious cycles of anxiety. He commented: 'It's beginning to make sense now. I wasn't reassured when I thought you were telling me that it was all in my mind, but now I understand what's happening'. He did dispute one factor in the formulation—he disagreed with his GP's suggestion that he suppressed emotion. He also added that, although he could accept the psychological explanation of his problem when he was somewhere he felt safe, i.e. the surgery or at home, his belief that he was having a heart attack was still very powerful when he was driving.

A case of obsessional–compulsive behaviour: Mr Oldham

The GP realized that Mr Oldham's problem was one which was anxiety related and reassured him that this was the case. He then suggested that the practice Community Psychiatric Nurse (CPN) be involved in helping Mr Oldham overcome his obsessional behaviour. The CPN had already been involved in psychological work and agreed to participate.

Collecting the relevant information

The CPN met Mr Oldham for an assessment session where he collected the following relevant information about the history of the problem.

Mr Oldham recalled being very relaxed as a youth. He had a good relationship with his parents, made friends easily, performed well at school, and felt that nothing really worried him very much. At the age of 18, he had to fight in the Second World War. There he experienced a number of traumatic incidents, one of which continued to haunt him. Towards the end of the war, a bomb exploded under a transport lorry which was carrying Mr Oldham's unit. He was the sole survivor, and witnessed the painful deaths of many of his friends. In addition to the psychological trauma, he received serious injuries, one of which left his right hand and wrist very weak.

When he left the army, he married and had three daughters. He had frequent nightmares about his experiences in the war and describes himself as being 'on edge' a good deal of the time. None the less, he lived a relatively untroubled life until his divorce 10 years ago. His separation was precipitated by the discovery that his wife was having an affair, which was a great shock to him. He said that during this time of distress he began to worry about things excessively, including security and safety issues. As his right hand and wrist were weak, he was never sure if he had really turned off a tap or twisted the door knob sufficiently, and his worrying became focused on these things. The immediate consequence of this preoccupation was that he spent less time thinking about his wife's decision to leave him.

Gradually, he seemed to adjust to his separation, and his obsessional behaviour reduced in frequency. A year later, when he had met his second wife, the checking behaviour remitted for several years. Eighteen months ago, he had been given a promotion at work, which meant that he carried much more responsibility. Although he was pleased to have been selected for promotion, he found his new position stressful and began to over-vigilant about checking documents and locks. This behaviour soon became part of his home life too. His wife tended to dismiss his difficulties as 'silly nonsense', and would refuse his requests the she ensure that things were safe in the house. This left him feeling embarrassed and even more anxious.

At the time of the assessment of Mr Oldham and his second wife were financially very comfortable, had no worries about their family, and both looked forward to Mr Oldham's forthcoming retirement.

Formulating Mr Oldham's problem

The CPN now was able to use these details to develop a formulation, which he discussed with Mr Oldham.

Vulnerability factors In trying to explain why Mr Oldham developed his particular problem, the CPN suggested that Mr Oldham's traumatic war experiences had increased his tendency to worry. He then pointed out that when faced with stress, Mr Oldham tended to focus his attention on issues other than the source of the stress. A further factor was the weakness in his wrist, which resulted in Mr Oldham doubting his ability to turn keys in locks or to twist knobs and switches effectively, thus giving him a focus for concern.

Precipitants His stress levels had recently increased as a result of his having to take on more responsibility at work. It is of note that this occurred at a time when he was preparing for another major life event, namely his retirement. The consequence of this stress was a reversion to his former coping strategy—checking safety.

Maintaining factors By giving in to the impulse to check, Mr Oldham could avoid the aversive sequelae of unpleasant physical symptoms and alarming and catastrophic thoughts. Therefore, he did succumb to the impulse, either by actually checking or transferring that responsibility to someone else. As long as he avoided the short-term physical and cognitive consequences of not checking he never learnt how to cope with the unpleasant experiences in an adaptive way. The long-term consequences were the chronicity of this behaviour, an erosion of his self-confidence, and a continuing failure to address his 'real' worries. A final factor was his wife's response to his need to check. By being critical of him, she further undermined his confidence and created more stress in him.

The CPN appreciated that any direct work with Mr Oldham could only be carried out at home, and not in his office. He also realized that Mrs Oldham could be involved in the treatment procedure but would need to understand more about the genesis and management of her husband's problem. By presenting the formulation to both Mr and Mrs Oldham, he was able to begin the process of education. Both felt that the formulation helped them to understand the checking behaviour. Mrs Oldham had actually known very little about her husband's war experience and his level of distress when he divorced his first wife, because he never talked about the incidents. However, she now said that she could see that he was not simply a 'weak, silly man', but someone who had a difficulty, which was understandable, given his history and current stress. She agreed that she could be more supportive.

A case of PTSD: Mr Thomas

The GP recognized that Mr Thomas' worsening mood was secondary to the recurring images of, and guilt surrounding, the road traffic accident. Although she had sometimes used antidepressant medication in conjunction with anxiety management work in the past, she decided not to prescribe until she had a fuller picture of Mr Thomas' problems. She then referred him to one of the practice counsellors for PTSD management.

Collecting the relevant information

In order to formulate Mr Thomas' problem, the practice counsellor took the following history in their first session: Mr Thomas was a successful script writer for the radio and had always enjoyed the freedom which it gave him. He married his girl-friend from college, who went on to become a solicitor. Four years ago, they had a son, Robert, and Mr Thomas happily assumed the role of primary caretaker, taking Robert to and from nursery school each day.

On the day of the accident, Mr Thomas drew up at a set of red lights, only yards from Robert's school. It was warm in the car, the cassette played soothing music and Mr Thomas gazed at the traffic-lights, thinking of the plot of his current script and not registering that they had changed to amber and red. Suddenly, he was jolted out of his day-dream by the sound of crunching metal as a large van ploughed into the side of his car, pushing it across the road. Witnesses reported that the van was going far too fast down a hill and the driver did not slow down as he reached the crossroad, perhaps anticipating that Mr Thomas would drive out of his way because the lights were changing to green.

The passenger side of the car, where Robert usually sat, was crushed and, as the car was moved sideways, a cyclist was trapped underneath. Mr Thomas could not open the door to get out, but through the broken window, he could see the bloody torso of a young woman whom he presumed dead.

An hour later, he was freed and rushed to hospital. It took longer to release the woman because her legs were so badly trapped and he later learnt that she was not dead but had been knocked unconscious. He also discovered that she might lose the use of her legs. After 24 hours, he was released from hospital with some lesions and a broken arm and ribs. Within a few months, he was physically well, the driver of the van had been prosecuted for dangerous driving and Mr Thomas was awarded significant compensation. The young woman, however, was not yet walking, although the neurological tests looked promising.

Recalling these details was extremely distressing for Mr Thomas and he and the counsellor took two or three breaks in the interview so that he could compose himself. In the following session, the counsellor discovered more about his background.

Mr Thomas was the only child of an academic couple. As expected, he gained an Oxbridge scholarship and studied English at University. He wanted to be a writer, but his parents disapproved. As he was fearful of their disapproval, he set high academic standards for himself and worked very hard to achieve them. He gained a first class degree and stayed on at his college to take a Masters degree. This was when he became involved with Carole, his first significant girl-friend. She was an undergraduate in law, much admired by his parents, and very supportive of his desire to write. With her support, he felt confident enough to send some of his work to the BBC and the scripts were accepted. His parents were still ambivalent about his writing. However, they were thrilled when their son married Carole and even more delighted when their grandson arrived.

The next few years were happy for the Thomas family, even though Mr Thomas' parents continued to be pessimistic about his career and overtly questioned the correctness of his taking on the role of Robert's caretaker. All this was tolerable until the accident, after which self-doubt took over. The counsellor asked him what it meant to him to be a less than perfect father, or to be an individual involved in a road traffic accident. He replied that 'It confirms my parents' view. I am a disappointment, no one is going to want to bother with me'.

Formulating Mr Thomas' problem

The counsellor was now able share her hypotheses concerning the onset and maintenance of Mr Thomas' difficulties.

Vulnerability factors Mr Thomas had grown up doubting his self-worth and trying to compensate by achieving high standards and pleasing his parents. His sense of worth, therefore, was based on his performance and not on positive feelings about himself.

Precipitants The shock of this road traffic accident was sufficient to evoke symptoms of distress in almost anyone. Mr Thomas was particularly vulnerable because the accident re-stimulated his self-doubts. Thus, he was much more likely to experience guilt and to ruminate on what he perceived as his weaknesses. The event also triggered his belief: 'I am a disappointment'.

Maintaining factors Typical of victims of trauma, Mr Thomas experienced 'flashbacks' and nightmares. These, in themselves, re-traumatized him, provoking distress which led him to conclude that he was never going to be free of the problem. His depressed mood added to his problems because the psychological and physical symptoms of depression are retarding. In addition, he was particularly vulnerable to depression and guilt because of low self-esteem which, once revitalized, exerted a powerful influence on his thinking. His problems were protracted by avoidance. This was in the form of overt avoidance of the feared situation where the accident happened and of driving. He employed subtle avoidance in the form of using only one 'safe' car and a single 'safe' driver. Thus he never resumed confidence that he could again drive in a variety of circumstances and vehicles.

When considering Mr Thomas' particular strengths and needs in treatment, the counsellor realized that a programme would have to be planned for success, so as to protect and build his self-esteem. She also felt that he had the advantages of a flexible timetable and his wife's understanding and support. She also realized that Mr Thomas was unaware of the natural consequences of trauma and needed to be educated about the phenomenon of PTSD.

A case of executive stress: Dr Evans

Dr Evans arrived late for her appointment with her GP, explaining that she'd been held up at work. She told the doctor about her episodes of disorientation and tinnitus and asked if he could prescribe something to stop this from happening. In the next breath, she asked if she was going mad.

The GP carried out a full investigation and concluded that there was no physical cause of her condition and suggested that she try to relax more.

Two weeks later, she returned to the surgery complaining that the problem was worsening: 'I never know when it is going to happen and it's happening more often. I can no longer commit myself to giving talks and there is an important conference in Paris in 12 week's time and I am supposed to represent my company and I don't think that I can. This is bound to damage my career and if I lose my job or get demoted, how do I pay the mortgage and the school fees? You have to give me something or send me to a specialist'.

The GP explained that he needed to talk things through with her before being able to make a decision about medication or referral to another agent. So, he arranged a double session with her the following day. She was not happy about this but she agreed to attend.

Collecting the relevant information

The GP discovered that Dr Evans was an only child. Her parents struggled financially and their marriage was always stormy. During some of the worst rows, she overheard her mother saying that she was leaving the family and Dr Evans was told that she would have to be fostered because the family could not afford to keep her. This threat was also used to discipline her.

Dr Evans did well at school and felt that this placated her parents who were always thrilled when she came top of the class.

She continued to work hard to achieve academic status, although she never felt that she was a 'natural'. At university, she met a postgraduate student called Mark, whom she felt was a 'natural academic'. They were married in her second year and then she went on to gain a first class degree. She stayed on to complete a doctorate and then embarked on an executive career while Mark remained in academia, largely supported by his wife's income. The marriage began to fail as they both devoted themselves to their careers and began to grow apart. She then discovered that she was pregnant with twins and she and her husband decided to stay together, hoping that the children would bind the marriage. As both were career oriented, they hired a nanny and later sent the children to prep and boarding school.

Unfortunately, the marriage continued to deteriorate and a divorce was precipitated when Dr Evans left Mark to live with her current husband—a colleague. The divorce was particularly acrimonious, with Mark arguing that his wife was 'an unfit, workaholic mother and adulteress'. The divorce proceedings lasted for 2 years, with Mark fighting for custody of the children and maintenance from his wife. They gained joint care and control of the twins and Dr Evans was obliged to pay maintenance. She saw the twins every other weekend and had them stay with her for half the school holidays. When asked about her first marriage, she said that she had put it all behind her.

She remarried 5 years ago and described this relationship as being more equal than her first marriage. Both she and her husband were ambitious, loved the excitement of business and had agreed not to have children. In fact, she was planning to have a hysterectomy because of the menorrhagia and dysmenorrhoea which had been worsening since the twins were born. In the 2 weeks before her first episode of dizziness, she had experienced her most extreme bout of heavy bleeding and menstrual clotting.

Formulating Dr Evan's problem

Her GP proposed the following explanation of Dr Evan's difficulties.

Vulnerability factors The GP suggested that the origin of her severe stress problem lay in her insecure and pressured childhood. He thought that Dr Evans had grown up with a sense of imminent danger, which elevated her stress levels. He also suggested that she held the belief that, in herself, she was not 'good enough' and her striving to compensate for this further contributed to her emotional strain.

Precipitants The particular incidents which had brought to fruition Dr Evans' distress, were her physical illness and an especially fraught return from Geneva. Her stress level at this time was further exacerbated by the cigarettes and coffee that she had taken on an empty stomach.

Maintaining factors Once her confidence had been undermined by her experience of disorientation, her fears of underachieving were re-stimulated. As a consequence, she had further episodes of self-doubt and performed less well in her job. To compensate, she pushed herself even harder and was soon caught up in a vicious cycle. To make matters worse, she misinterpreted her experience as an early sign of madness which, again, elevated her anxieties and brought on the distressing symptoms. Finally, her lifelong traits of impatience and pushing herself to the limit, only made the problem more difficult to tackle by ensuring that her arousal levels were always high.

The GP realized that Dr. Evans was now suffering the consequences of her life-style, her personality type, and her physical condition. Although he was optimistic that the medical profession could ease her menstrual problems, he was concerned that she would not be willing to alter her life-style or her approach to life. He shared his formulation with Dr Evans, and sure enough, she resisted change.

'My work is me; it is my excitement and fulfilment. You can't ask me to lose that' she protested. This gave her doctor the opportunity to explain that she would not have to sacrifice her job and her outlook, but that therapy would aim to help her to recognize the early signs of excess stress and teach her how to pull herself back from the brink. She remained unconvinced that such a procedure would not endanger her career. So, the GP suggested that consider this a trial which would enable them to discover if stress management would be helpful in her case. If, after 10 sessions, she remained unconvinced, she could always revert to her previous way of working.

Dealing with problems

Following the initial assessment the presenting problem may seem too chronic or complex to be dealt with using a short-term and very simple cognitive–behavioural approach. If this is the case, consider referring the client to a clinical psychologist, psychiatrist, or other appropriate agent. Often, the complexity of a problem is not apparent until treatment is underway. This does not prevent the subsequent involvement of another therapist, as progress can be reviewed at the end of a contracted number of sessions, with a view to considering referral. Do not be afraid of referring to another agent; it is not an indication of failure on your part, but would suggest that the short-term stress management approach is not suited to your client. It is then best for the client if responsibility for treatment is transferred as soon as possible, in the way that you might transfer a patient to a specialist in cardiology or orthopaedics.

7 *Control*

The therapist's object in teaching AMT is to ensure that a client develops the capacity to cope effectively with stress. It is crucial that the therapist select the right control techniques for each client, with regard to that person's training needs and resources.

Meeting client needs: which technique to choose

The choice of coping skills to be used depends on the presenting problem, the particular strengths and needs of the client, and the client's successes or failures. Making the right choice depends on the therapist having a good formulation of the problem to work from and being flexible in personalizing the management plan.

When to use relaxation training

Most AMT therapists begin treatment with relaxation training because it is invariably useful, readily learnt, and has a good deal of credibility for the client. Relaxation can provide relief from both physical and mental tension, gives the client experience in controlling the tension, and provides specific skills that can be applied to the anxiety-provoking situations which will have to be faced during treatment.

Relaxation training is particularly helpful for those people who complain of specific aches and pains, of general tension, or of an inability to relax. Forms of relaxation training vary and include yoga, meditation, PMR training, and hypnotically induced relaxation. The training can be undertaken by the therapist, or it might be reasonable to suggest that the individual join a relaxation group or take up yoga, for example.

If it is decided to teach relaxation training, remember that the objective is to guide the client through a series of progressively shorter exercises until he or she has a skill which can be applied as needed. The stages in developing relaxation skills are rather like those in learning a language: one begins with the vocabulary which is fundamental but of limited application; one then moves on to developing grammar which makes the vocabulary of greater use; finally, one covers semantics, thus creating a meaningful and useful skill.

In teaching relaxation skills, you might begin with a lengthy and highly structured exercise like Jacobsen's PMR exercise, followed by a shorter progressive exercise. Then, you could direct the client to brief regimen such as Benson's relaxation routine and finally move on to the very brief, cued relaxation techniques. You can increase compliance by preparing a series of instruction tapes for clients. Instructions for making your own tapes are printed in Appendix 6 of this book.

When to teach controlled breathing

As increased respiration rate is a common symptom of anxiety, and as most people find the effects of hyperventilation unpleasant and often frightening, it is helpful to teach good breathing techniques as a matter of course. It is certainly advisable to teach controlled breathing if your client experiences panic attacks and you suspect that overbreathing is an important factor in the development of the panic. The instructions for controlled breathing are detailed in Chapter 12, which is concerned with working with your client.

When to teach thought management

If a client identifies distressing thoughts or fantasies as part of the problem anxiety, then your approach should involve thought management. It has been noted that the more anxious the person, the less easily the complex strategies are applied. So, distraction through physical activity would be appropriate for the extremely anxious, while the less stressed client could be instructed in more mentally demanding techniques such as creative thinking. In order to ensure that a client has recourse to distraction techniques when stressed, she or he needs to have built up and practised a repertoire of distracting activities and mental diversions.

The decision to use distraction or challenging as a coping method depends, to some extent, on the person's ability to adopt the more demanding technique of challenging. The ability to use this approach is often established through trial and is likely to be apparent within a few sessions. As was mentioned earlier, distraction should not be used as an avoidance strategy.

When to introduce panic management

The indications for this are the symptoms of panic attack which were outlined in Chapter 1. Where hyperventilation seems to be a major part of the problem, emphasis should be on teaching controlled breathing (see Chapter 12). In addition, anyone complaining of panic attack should be thoroughly rehearsed in control techniques so that they can use the strategies, almost automatically, as they are needed.

Combining the techniques

Often, maximum benefits are derived from AMT when coping strategies are used in combination. For example, relaxation can be coupled with imagery, or controlled breathing with distraction. Anxiety management techniques can also be supplemented by other skills training which might be available elsewhere, such as social skills or assertiveness training for the socially phobic time management training for the person whose stress is exacerbated by poor organization.

Building on client strengths

When developing a treatment plan, use your knowledge of your client's resources. For example, involve a supportive spouse in a relaxation programme if this helps your client to practice more regularly, or involve a relative in carrying out problem-solving exercises. If your client has a social phobia and is a car owner, you could realistically plan goals which involved travelling to social organizations which would otherwise be inaccessible.

There will also be personal resources to consider. If a person has practised meditation, then you could expect her or him to respond quickly to relaxation training and perhaps distraction. Someone else might have enjoyed sport in the past and would be easily encouraged to developed physical exercise as distraction technique.

8 *Dealing with avoidance*

A client who has successfully developed some confidence in combating the symptoms of fear, can be encouraged to use the same skills in anxiety-provoking situations. At this stage of therapy, the therapist and client work together very closely. The setting of targets and grading of tasks is a collaborative activity which gradually becomes the sole work of the client. The target is whatever she or he fears; a task is a graded step on the way to a target.

Setting the target

In setting targets, first ask your client to list the situations or objects which are anxiety provoking now but which she or he expects to be able to face in the future. These goals of therapy must be concrete, specific, and realistic. Initially, you will probably have to help your client to define the target(s) clearly. When you and your client have arrived at a list of well-defined goals, these should be arranged in a hierarchy of difficulty or urgency.

As your client acquires the skills of target setting you can gradually transfer that responsibility to him or her.

Grading the task

Targets are approached in carefully worked out stages or tasks. The essential features of tasks are that they are concrete, observable or measurable, realistic, and graded according to difficulty. The aim at this stage of AMT is to restore the lost confidence of the client by helping that person to build on a series of successful experiences. The risk of failure really must be avoided. The most common reason for an unsuccessful experience is that someone has attempted too much too soon.

In the early stages of therapy give your client help in planning a series of small, very specific tasks of increasing difficulty. Do not be afraid of being flexible and encouraging your client to devise contingency plans in case the planned task turns out to be impossible to execute. As therapy proceeds you can expect your client to do more of the planning, but supervision is necessary to ensure that any plans are realistic. If your client cannot manage a task, this is not a failure, it is simply that the step which was taken was too difficult for that person at that time. If this happens, break the step down further and try again. It is better to achieve something in many small steps than risk not coping at any stage.

Practising

Practise is the most important part of the treatment, because it is by rehearsing in stressful situations that fear is overcome. To be effective, practice in the feared situation must be continued until the associated anxiety has died away. This exposure work is best carried out in conjunction with other anxiety-reducing techniques such as relaxation and thought management.

Exposure is not effective unless it is repeated, so set homework which involves frequent and regular practice. It is helpful for the client to keep a record of progress, which will then provide useful information for both him or her and therapist each time homework is reviewed. If favourable progress is documented, this record can positively reinforce practice. It is not uncommon for people to become disappointed because they underrate their achievements but a written account of progress can help to minimize disappointment which is based on subjective and distorted recall. Your client may need to be encouraged to be objective about progress, to recognize achievements, and to praise success.

A final point is that you may wish to involve friends and relatives in helping the client follow the programme.

Independence

As the client becomes more experienced in stress control, and more skilful in problem solving and planning, the frequency of appointments can be reduced so that the client works with less supervision and learns to cope independently of the therapist.

Dealing with problems

There are, of course, set-backs from time to time. When this happens, it is likely that too difficult a task has been attempted, perhaps in a bout of enthusiasm or just through careless planning. Alternatively, someone might simply have had a 'bad day' because of fatigue, illness, or stress. If your client has achieved a task on a previous day, it is particularly demoralizing when it is not successfully repeated. Try to prepare your client for disappointment and encourage a realistic appraisal of personal limitations, which may indeed vary from day to day. Emphasize that set-backs are expected and that one should not be discouraged and give up prematurely. Try to help your client realize that more can be learnt about personal limitations and resources through having set-backs.

9 *Self-management and ending therapy*

The goal of the therapist is to ensure that the client has a working knowledge of anxiety management techniques. It might be some time before the client has practised these sufficiently to feel confident and trouble free. However, the therapist should not be afraid of stopping AMT before a client is fully confident. Often, confidence only grows through independent practice.

Deciding when your client can cope alone

It is important to review your client's progress regularly, using both verbal report and evidence from diaries. The crucial decision to be made is whether the person has the knowledge, skills, and confidence to cope without your guidance. In general, support can be withdrawn when the client understands the maintaining factors in her or his problem, is capable of practising stress management and can problem solve and plan appropriately, and is confident enough to confront difficult situations.

It is very important to discourage dependency. When you are sure that the client has the ability to cope alone, be sensitive but firm about finishing AMT.

How to prepare your client

It is always best to prepare your client for the end of your intervention well in advance, as he or she might need time to adjust to the termination of therapy. If therapy can only be given for a limited time, state this at the outset and fix a termination date.

When working within the contract system, inform the client that, at the end of each period, progress will be reviewed with a view to ending this treatment, if this is appropriate. Whether working with or without the contract arrangement, once a decision has been made that the client can cope alone, specify a finite number of AMT sessions before the intervention ends.

Blueprinting

Blueprinting is the process of identifying personal problem areas or times of vulnerability and then generating solutions to these potentially difficult situations. The solutions will reflect a client's adaptive coping skills and resources available. At this stage, your client should be able to identify problem areas and solutions with only minimal help from you.

You can best prepare your client for long-term coping if you have anticipated future difficulties and discovered what resources are going to be available. By the end of therapy you should be familiar with your client's weaknesses and needs. Perhaps she or he has a tendency to be over-ambitious or to use alcohol in a crisis, in which case alternative and more helpful behaviours should be explored and rehearsed. Maybe your client has ongoing marital problems or poor social skills and perhaps there are resources available such as marriage guidance counselling, local support groups, or social skills training classes to which she or he could be directed.

Arranging a follow-up appointment

It is useful, although not compulsory, to arrange to see your client a month or two after you have finished the course in AMT. A distant appointment can be reassuring for nervous or dependent people, while affording them the real apportunity to practise alone. This period of independence often consolidates skills and when this happens, self-confidence improves. In addition, difficulties experienced during this period can be reviewed and help can be given where appropriate. Finally, follow-up appointments permit the therapist to evaluate the efficacy of treatment in a real-life setting.

It is necessary to indicate that the follow-up is a review session and not the beginning of another course of therapy. Of course, should you feel that your client needs further help, you can consider setting a contract for another series of sessions or referring him or her to another agent.

10 *Summary of Part II: Preparatory notes for the therapist*

Summary of Chapter 6: Anxiety

The assessment session(s) comprise(s) the following:

(1) Presenting problem
- (i) client's own description;
- (ii) example of a recent incident: look for
  - (a) somatic, cognitive, and behavioural factors,
  - (b) antecedents and consequents;
- (iii) duration, frequency, severity;
- (iv) events or situations which exacerbate or ameliorate the problem.

(2) History of the problem
- (i) predisposing factors—personal and family factors;
- (ii) onset-related factors;
- (iii) course.

(3) Current coping methods
- (i) adaptive;
- (ii) maladaptive.

(4) Relevant investigations
- (i) psychological;
- (ii) medical.

(5) Previous treatment
- (i) psychological;
- (ii) other.

(6) Current involvement of other agencies.

(7) Current medication
including caffeine, alcohol, cigarettes, self-medication.

(8) Client expectations of treatment and motivation to change.

(9) Personal targets of change: detailed and specific.

(10) Other relevant details
  - (i) mood
  - (ii) social, family, marital situation (including available social support)
  - (iii) employment details.

This information will enable you to generate a formulation and personalized intervention plan.

Diary keeping can be used to supplement the assessment.

Contracts are useful in the organization of appointments.

Summary of Chapter 7: Control

Use your formulation to establish treatments needs, as shown below

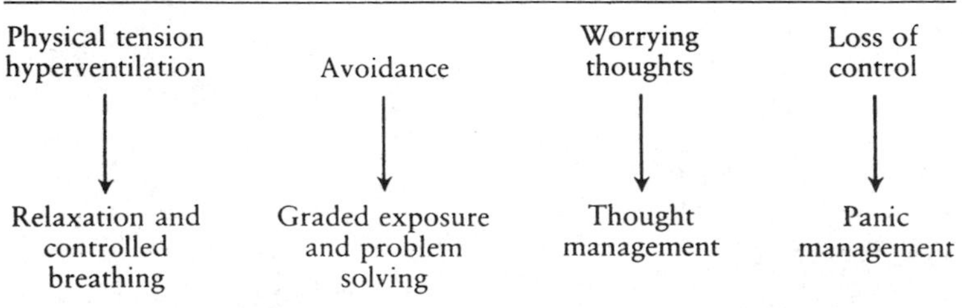

Modify your approach according to your client's resources.

Summary of Chapter 8: Dealing with avoidance

In the early stages of therapy:

(1) work closely with your client in target setting and grading tasks;

(2) check that targets are realistic, measurable, concrete, specific, and graded for success;

(3) set homework of repeated practice.

As therapy proceeds:

(4) reduce active role of therapist;

(5) reduce frequency of appointments;

(6) maintain good supervision.

Summary of Chapter 9: Self-management and ending therapy

(1) Assess progress and decide if termination is appropriate.

(2) Anticipate your client's long-term needs: blueprint.

(3) Discourage dependency.

(4) Make a definite follow-up appointment.

PART III

Working with your client

11 *Anxiety*

Once a decision has been made to offer stress management, the therapist has two objectives. First, to present the option for treatment, with its rationale; and secondly, to establish a collaborative relationship with the client, introducing the concept of homework.

Presenting the client with the option for treatment

This is usefully achieved by discussing your formulation of the problem to your client. The formulation explains why you believe anxiety to be the problem and the management approach which you could adopt, while emphasizing that the client would have to learn self-help skills to control the symptoms.

Other advantages of presenting the formulation are that it introduces the psychological model of the development of problem anxiety and the client can begin to collaborate with the therapist in commenting upon and perhaps modifying the formulation.

The decision to take up this option of treatment lies, of course, with the client. In accepting therapy, people should realize that most of the 'work' is in the form of homework.

Presenting the client with the rationale behind AMT

First, make sure your client understands how normal anxiety develops and how this might become a problem. Explain that the feelings of anxiety can be controlled, though they will never go away. Presentation of the stress cycle in the development of tension is useful at this point. To help your client remember this information, give her or him information about anxiety (see Client Information Sheet 1 on pp. 96).

Next, reassure your client that one can learn to identify feelings of stress and develop effective ways of coping with them. Outline the procedure whereby skills are learned through practice outside the sessions.

Emphasize that the goal of treatment is not the elimination of anxiety, but the acquisition of skills to control and take charge of unpleasant feelings.

Introduce your formulation of the problem to your client, and get feedback on its accuracy by asking questions such as 'Have I missed anything out?', 'Does this fit with your view of your problem?', Correct me if I am wrong.'

It is important that you make it clear to your client that you are aware that he or she is currently experiencing very unpleasant feelings. Emphasize, however, that therapy will focus on learning techniques to control them, rather than spending time exploring the experiences.

Establishing a good working relationship

Enlist your clients as collaborators right from the start. It is essential that they appreciate that the therapeutic relationship will be a working partnership and that their role will not be passive. At this stage your success in engaging someone in therapy will depend largely on their understanding and remembering of information and their level of compliance.

Understanding and remembering information is affected by a number of factors. People fail to understand information which is too difficult or sophisticated, if they have a poor elementary knowledge of the subject, or if their opinions are biased by misconceptions. They do not remember information if presented with too much, if it is presented in a poorly organized fashion, or if it is too difficult or sophisticated.

You can help your client by giving as few instructions as possible, so try to think ahead and decide which are most pertinent. Bear in mind that people remember best those instructions which are given first or emphasized, and that specific instructions are remembered better than management rules, and management rules better than general information.

Present the information thoughtfully and remember to check the client's understanding of what you have said as you go along. You could try saying something like: 'We have covered quite a bit of information in terms of exploring your problem; now it might be useful if you try to recall what we've discussed', 'At this point, imagine I am the one learning about my problem—how would you explain it to me? Do not be afraid of repeating yourself during a session: this will serve to reinforce a point. As people tend to forget over half of the information they are given, it is essential to provide your client with written information (see Client Information Sheet 1, on pp. 96), so that an informed decision about treatment can be made.

Compliance with treatment is essential. Non-compliance has been shown to be associated with dissatisfaction in the recipient, complex regimens, treatment of long duration, and expensive therapies. To offset this, the therapist should consider how a client feels about therapy, keep any regimen as simple as possible, make it clear that the person will be supported throughout the treatment, and be sensitive to financial limitations and try to tailor treatment plans accordingly.

Where possible, try to anticipate situations which might jeopardize compliance by asking questions like, 'I wonder what problems you foresee?' This will give you an opportunity to deal with issues like social embarrassment and forgetfulness before they hinder treatment. Giving a specific appointment with an identified therapist has also been shown to increase compliance, so remember to make a repeat appointment rather than relying on the client to initiate contact again.

Setting homework

You should make sure that your client realizes that homework tasks are fundamental to the success of treatment. The function of your meeting is to structure and plan the work to be done outside the session. In the sessions, the therapist works out very clear and specific tasks with the client.

Homework should begin with the first appointment. The first task is usually, but not necessarily, diary keeping (see Diaries 1–3 in Appendix 7). Homework should be reviewed each session, even if this means working through quite a few detailed diaries. If your client has done an assignment, it is important not to neglect it. If, however, you do find that your client consistently brings in an excessive amount of self-monitoring data, you could ask them to summarize and identify the main themes before each session. This will make your task easier and might also help a disorganized client to learn to précis and prioritize—a skill which is necessary if she or he is to learn to manage independently.

Client information sheet 1: **What is anxiety?**

Anxiety is common. It is the normal response to danger or stress and only becomes a problem when it is out of proportion to a situation or if it goes on too long.

Anxiety is not damaging. It cannot cause physical or mental harm, but it can make life difficult when it gets out of control. When it does, thinking and doing, and even the most simple things can become an enormous strain.

Anxiety is crucial to our survival because it prepares us for coping with stress. It is the trigger for hormonal changes in our bodies which enables us to cope with danger by preparing us for *fight or flight*. This produces many of the *bodily feelings* which we can associate with anxiety, such as:

tense muscles
racing heart
rapid breathing
sweating

When we are anxious, our t*hinking patterns* also change, the most common being: preoccupation with the problem and not noticing other things.

In the short-term, these changes are helpful because our bodies are prepared for physical action and our minds become focused on the immediate problem. The changes evolved to be an immediate response to stress which was switched off as soon as the danger passed. If these reactions are not switched off, the bodily sensations become more unpleasant, and result in:

muscular pains
sweating profusely
difficulty breathing
pounding heart
weak legs
trembling
churning stomach.

Thinking will become more focused on worrying:

always fearing the worst
thinking negatively
worrying that the problem is permanent
believing the problem is physical.

At this point, anxiety itself can become distressing and when this happens, a cycle is set up and the worrying can easily get out of control.

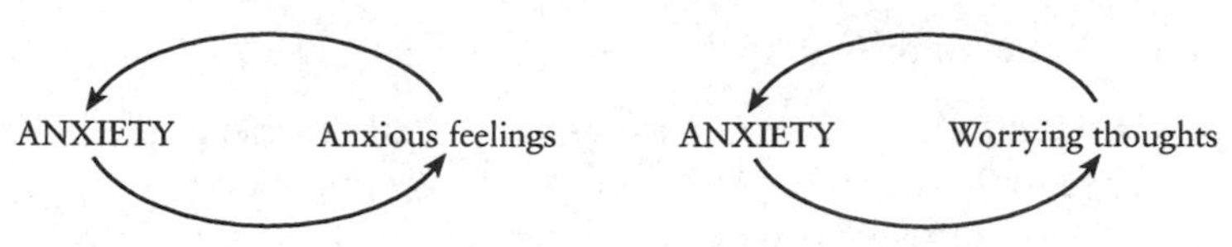

At times of stress, our *behaviour* can change, too:

fidgeting	nail biting
increased drinking	running away
avoiding situations	smoking more
rushing around	comfort eating

The most common response to fear is running away, but the relief from avoiding is only temporary, then the situation becomes increasingly difficult to face and another cycle develops.

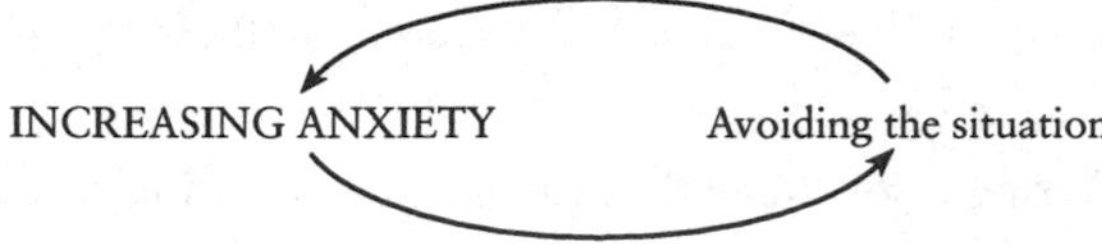

What can I do to control my anxiety?

You can learn to break these cycles of increasing anxiety by developing practical ways of overcoming the unpleasant symptoms. Three methods are particularly useful:

1. Learning to relax.
2. Learning to control distressing thoughts.
3. Learning to face the fear.

By using these approaches, the unhelpful cycles described above can be brought under control. These methods of control do not necessarily come naturally. They are skills which need to be learned through regular practice. Developing the skill of anxiety management is rather like learning to play a musical instrument or learning another language: if you want to do it properly, you have to find time to practice. With practice, you will develop coping skills to use whenever you are under stress or anxious. You will then be able to control unpleasant feelings and to face difficult situations.

Get to know your anxiety

Anxiety is different for each of us. We do not all experience the same bodily sensations, each of us has our own worrying thoughts and we each behave differently when under stress. In addition, triggers for anxiety vary from person to person. Before you can begin to learn how to manage anxiety, you must understand your own problem. You can do this by keeping a record of when you are anxious and then noting how you feel, think, and what you do. It is also useful to make an estimate of how anxious you feel in different situations by rating your stress levels on a 0–10 scale of increasing anxiety. Keep a note of your anxiety for 1 or 2 weeks and then look back over your entries. You should find that you can answer the questions:

What things or situations trigger *my* anxiety?

What are *my* bodily feelings and *my* anxious thoughts when I am stressed?

What differing levels of anxiety do different situations cause?

What do I tend to do when I am anxious?

What helps *me* to cope with my anxiety?

Get to know your coping skills

The last question is particularly important as you must distinguish between the coping strategies which are helpful in the long run and those which might make you fell better in the short-term, but are not helpful over time.

Long-term coping strategies would include: taking exercise, doing some yoga, or talking to yourself in a soothing, constructive way. All of these are beneficial immediately and in the long-term.

Short-term coping would include: relying on tranquillizers or alcohol, avoiding difficult situations, or scolding yourself. Be especially careful not to turn to stimulants when you are under stress as they will increase the unpleasant bodily symptoms and make coping more difficult. The sorts of stimulants which you might use are alcohol, cigarettes, chocolate, chocolate drinks, coffee, cola drinks, or tea.

Don't feel that you have to abandon your short-term coping strategies at once: this can be too alarming a prospect. Instead, think how you might begin to integrate more helpful coping strategies into you repertoire of techniques.

When you are familiar with your own problem anxiety, you will be ready to develop a new set of coping strategies to suit *your* needs.

Dealing with problems

Somaticizing of symptoms

Some people find it difficult to accept that a problem is not of organic origin. When this is the case, you could try either of two approaches.

First, you can suggest to your client that, in order to rule out a psychological diagnosis, you first need to try out a psychological approach to discover if it works in your client's case. If, after a genuine trial of psychological intervention, there has been no improvement you might re-evaluate the problem. You should emphasize that this experimental approach is only viable if the psychological methods are applied with sincerity on the part of your client.

Secondly, you can suggest that the client keeps a diary of physical complaints (see Diary 3 in Appendix 7) over several days. Patterns are likely to emerge which are linked to psychological variables, for examples a mother's headaches might be more frequent or more severe around the time that her children come home from school. This information would suggest that the condition was not physical, but stress related.

Non-compliance

If your client does not fully engage in therapy, and does not attend appointments or carry out homework tasks, then you should consider referring that person to another agent. The reasons for apparent non-compliance are many: low self-esteem giving rise to hopelessness, fear of failure causing avoidance, a very powerful belief in a physiological cause of the problem and so on. It is possible that your client has a psychological block to self-help and will need a skilled therapist's help to overcome this. It is often better to involve the specialist early rather than establish an unsuccessful working pattern with your client.

12 *Control*

When your client has accepted a psychological formulation of the problem, and has agreed to AMT, your task as the therapist is to help that person develop the appropriate coping skills.

Preparing your client

Remind your client that the goal of treatment is not the elimination of anxiety, but learning the skills necessary to take charge of the unpleasant feelings. Emphasize that stress control is always easier when anxiety is in this early stages, and thus the client will learn to use the feelings or tension as a cue for immediate action.

Explain that a combination of techniques may be appropriate, but that these will be learnt and practised as individual strategies. At first they will be practised only at times of low anxiety. Later, they will be introduced into situations which provoke tension. When preparing your client, introduce the concept of diary keeping, using the diaries in Appendix 7 if you wish.

Introducing diary keeping

As retrospective data are unreliable, emphasize the importance of collecting information during the period of stress. After the initial contact, the therapist can state, 'This was a useful discussion and I have a reasonable idea of your experiences. However, we will get an even better understanding of the nature of your problem if you record what you feel (or think, or do) at the actual time of stress. Everyone's anxiety is different, and we need to know more about your particular experience as it happens'.

Explain that information from the diary will help you to establish patterns of anxiety symptoms. From these you can start to make predictions about the problem and eventually plan to take control of unpleasant feelings. Read through the diary, checking that your client understands how to use the anxiety rating scale and realizes what information is required. You can ask him or her to practise by rating anxiety during the session. You can then see for yourself if the procedure has been understood. Also ask, 'What problems do you foresee?' so that you can pre-empt them.

Introducing relaxation training

First, explain the role of tension in producing or exacerbating symptoms of anxiety, and how relaxation can offset these. Then check that your client relates her or his own problem to this. Emphasize that relaxation is a self-help skill which needs regular practice—at least daily. You can use an analogy, such as having to learn basic vocabulary in order to speak another language, or to practise scales in order to play the piano well. Convey the message that the amount of gain is directly related to the amount of practice. Remind your client of the essential elements of successful relaxation: a quiet environment, a comfortable position, a mental image to promote tranquillity, passive attitude (Benson 1975).

Go through the procedure given in Client Information Sheet 2 on page 103. This sheet contains practical suggestions and a series of graded exercises of decreasing length. The first exercise is Jacobsen's PMR, a lengthy and thorough exercise. Explain that once this routine is mastered, your client will move on to increasingly shorter exercises until she or he has acquired the skill to relax quite swiftly and at will.

When your client reports complete relaxation at the end of an exercise, you will know that it is time to move to a shorter regimen. These shorter routines are also printed on the information sheet.

Always explain that the exercises might feel strange at first and might be difficult and time-consuming to carry out. Emphasize that the relaxation process becomes more comfortable, quicker, and easier with practice.

Set homework, specifying how often the exercises are to be done. In consultation with the client, decide the best time of day and place for the work. Try to pre-empt reasons for not practising relaxation. Remember to invite questions and to provide a relaxation training tape, if necessary.

Client information sheet 2: **Controlling bodily feeling of anxiety**

Relaxation

Whenever we are anxious or stressed, the muscles in our bodies tense. When muscles become too tense, we experience uncomfortable sensations such as, headache, stiff neck, painful shoulders, tight chest, difficulty in breathing, trembling, tingling hands and face, back pain … and more.

These sensations can make us even more anxious, which in turn, increases muscular tension. The result is a spiral of worsening tension which can become increasingly distressing.

The most effective way of controlling bodily tension is by relaxing. Relaxing isn't just a matter of sitting in front of the television or having a hobby (although these recreations are important too), you need to develop a skill which will enable you to reduce unnecessary physical tension whenever you need to. You can then use this skill to relieve anxiety and the associated unpleasant bodily sensations in a variety of situations. Furthermore, when your body is free of tension, your mind tends to be relaxed, too.

The ability to relax does not always come easily, it is a skill which has to be learned by progressing through a series of structured exercises. The following routines are designed to help you to learn to relax in a series of steps. The first two are quite long and you may find that taped instructions are helpful.

General guide-lines

- Before doing the exercise, decide when you will practice, and try to keep to this time each day so that you develop a routine.
- Practice two or three times a day: the more you practice the more easily you will be able to relax.
- Choose somewhere quiet to exercise where no one will disturb you. Do not attempt your exercise if you are hungry or have just eaten; or if the room is too hot or too chilly. This will make it more difficult to relax.

- Start the exercise by lying down in a comfortable position, wearing comfortable clothes. Later, you can also practice relaxation while you are sitting or standing.
- Try to adopt a passive attitude, i.e. do not worry about your performance or whether you are successfully relaxing. Just have a go and let it happen.
- *Breathing*: try to breathe through your nose, filling your lungs completely so that you feel your stomach muscles stretch. Breathe slowly and regularly and do not take a lot of quick, deep breaths as this can make you fell dizzy or faint. If you place your hands on your stomach, you will feel movement there if you are breathing properly. Try this out before you exercise to make sure that you are used to the feeling.
- Record your progress because you need to know if relaxation is working for you. Expect day-to-day variation in your ability to relax—we all have days when it comes easily and other days when relaxation is more difficult.

The exercises

As you will not be able to relax *and* read the instructions very easily, first read through all the exercises to get familiar with the routines. Then you can start to work through the four exercises, which get progressively shorter. When you are able to relax using the first exercise, move on to the second, then the third and finally learn exercise four, which is a rapid relaxation routine. This whole process should be done over several weeks. The precise length of time needed will vary from person to person. Only move to the next exercise when you can *really* relax at the end of a routine as there is nothing to be gained by rushing through the programme.

1. Progressive muscular relaxation

This first exercise will help you to distinguish between tense and relaxed muscles, so that you can recognize when you are tense and then relax in response to this. The basic movement which you use at every stage of the exercise is as follows. First, tense your muscles gently, really concentrating on the feelings of tension and strain. Hold this for about 5 seconds and then let go of the tension for 10–15 seconds. Discover how your muscles feel when you relax them. Focus on the sensations in the different parts of your body. The relaxation exercise involves doing this for all parts of your body.

The procedure

- FEET Pull your toes back, tense the muscles in your feet. Relax and repeat.
- LEGS Straighten your legs, point your toes towards your face. Relax and repeat.
- ABDOMEN Tense your stomach muscles by pulling them in and up. Relax and repeat.
- BACK Arch your back. Relax and repeat.
- SHOULDERS AND NECK Shrug your shoulders firmly, bringing them up and in. Press your head back. Relax and repeat.
- ARMS Stretch out your arms and hand. Relax and repeat.
- FACE Tense your forehead and jaw. Lower your eyebrows and bite. Relax and repeat.
- WHOLE BODY Tense your entire body. Feet, legs, abdomen, back, shoulders and neck, arms, and face. Hold the tension for a few seconds. Relax and repeat.

NOTE: Breathe slowly and regularly between each stage in the procedure and during the exercise.

If, when you reach the end of the routine, you still feel tense, then go through it again. If only parts of your body feel tense, repeat the exercise just in those areas. When you have finished the exercise, spend a few moments relaxing your mind. Think about something restful—whatever scene or image works best for you. Breathe slowly through your nose, filling your lungs completely. Continue for a minute or two, then open your eyes. Do not stand up straight away, and when you are ready, move *slowly* and stretch *gently*.

2. Shortened progressive relaxation

You can shorten the routine by missing out the 'tense' stage, going through the routine by systematically relaxing the different muscle groups. When you can do this, you can adapt the routine to use at other times and in other places. For example, you might try the exercise sitting down rather than in a lying position; or you might move from a quiet bedroom to the living area, which is not so peaceful. In this way, you will be learning to relax in a range of environments, which is what you need for real life coping.

3. Simple relaxation routine

This is an even shorter exercise which you can practice as you become more experienced at achieving the relaxed state. For this exercise, you will need to imagine a soothing, restful mental image to use during the routine. Your mental image will help you to relax even more effectively. It can be:

- A sound or word which you find relaxing, such as the word 'calm' or the sound of the sea.
- A particular object which is restful, perhaps a picture or an ornament which you particularly like.
- A scene which you find calming, such as a quiet country scene or a deserted beach.

The procedure

- Sit in a comfortable position with your eyes closed. Imagine your body growing heavier and more relaxed.
- Breathe through your nose and become aware of your breathing. As you breathe out, think about your mental image, while breathing easily and naturally.
- Don't worry whether or not you are good at the exercise, simply let go of your tensions and relax at your own pace. Distracting thoughts will probably come into your mind. Don't worry about this and don't dwell on them, simply return to thinking about your mental image or your breathing pattern.

- Keep this going for 10–20 minutes. When you finish, sit quietly with your eyes closed for a few moments, and then sit with your eyes open. Don't stand up or begin moving around quickly.

With practice, you will be able to respond to stress by relaxing, almost automatically.

4. Cued relaxation

When you are able to relax using exercises 1–3, you can begin to use your relaxation skills throughout the day and not just your designated 'relaxation time'. In this way, you will gain the ability to relax at will whenever it is necessary. All you need is something which will catch your eye regularly and remind you to:

- drop your shoulders;
- untense the muscles in your body;
- check your breathing;
- relax.

As a cue, or reminder, you might use a small, coloured spot on your watch or something else which you look at regularly during the day. Every time you see the cue, you will be reminded to relax and you will be practising your relaxation skills several times a day. There are all sorts of cues which you might use—work out what catches your eye frequently and use this as a reminder.

With time and regular practice, relaxation will become a way of life. You are bound to experience stress, anxiety and tension at some time—this is normal—but you will now have a better awareness of your tension and the skills to bring it under control.

Dealing with problems

'I get peculiar feelings when I do the exercises': Remind your client that it is usual to feel strange when carrying out a novel task and give reassurance that the odd sensations will disappear. Check that your client is not hyperventilating during the exercise, or standing up too quickly after completing the routine, or practising when too hungry or too full, as these can cause unpleasant reactions.

'I get cramps': Advise your client not to use too cold a room and not to tense muscles too vigorously. Rubbing the affected muscle can ease the cramp, and then the exercise can be completed—gently!

'I fall asleep': When this happens and it is not the object of the exercise, you can suggest sitting, rather than lying down, for the exercise, as this might be less conducive to sleep. Resting an elbow on the arm of the chair can help because it may slip off and awaken the sleeper.

'I get intruding, worrying thoughts': As this is quite normal, you can reassure your client that it is not a serious problem and that the thoughts will disappear if they are not dwelt upon. The best thing to do is to accept the intrusion of the thoughts but to return to focusing on the relaxation exercise. If your client tries *not* to think about the thoughts, it will be impossible to think of anything else.

'I don't feel relaxed': The most important thing is not to try too hard. Anyone who is determined to relax will not be able to un-tense themselves very easily. Remind your client of the need to adopt a passive attitude, and give reassurance that relaxation is a skill which will improve with practice. In addition, check that the exercise is being carried out in a comfortable environment.

'I can't let go and simply relax': Some individuals do have difficulty in 'letting go'. Sometimes this is because the feeling of muscular relaxation is unfamiliar and seems unpleasant, sometimes the experience is unwelcome because it signifies something unacceptable to the client, such as sloth or vulnerability. If this is an obstacle to relaxation training, you could suggest beginning with the brief exercise and gradually build up to the lengthy ones.

Introducing controlled breathing

Should you decide to focus on breathing, you will need to do this in two stages. First explain the rationale and then introduce the technique.

Explain the origin of overbreathing and its consequences, reassuring your client that no physical harm results from hyperventilation. You can use Client Information Sheet 3 on page 110 to supplement your discussion.

The practical exercise which is detailed below was developed by Clark *et al.* (1985) to help people recognize and then control the symptoms of hyperventilation. They suggest that you ask the client to carry out a practical session of overbreathing before you introduce the rationale for controlled respiration. When your client understands the link between overbreathing and unpleasant physical sensations, you can teach controlled respiration as an anxiety management technique.

The hyperventilation exercise

Voluntary hyperventilation

An optional, diagnostic stage to establish whether the symptoms described are the result of hyperventilation. Clients are required to breathe deeply and quickly (40–60 breaths per minute) through the mouth and nose, for two minutes. They are always reassured that the unpleasant feelings can be offset by breathing into a paper bag which is made available. They are asked to list the symptoms which are experienced during overbreathing and then to state how similar these are to the feelings of anxiety.

Explanation

Next, they are told of the association between overbreathing and feelings of anxiety, and how the feelings may get out of control.

Training in slow breathing

The aim of this stage is to teach clients a pattern of respiration which is incompatible with hyperventilation, and which can be used in controlling anxiety. Clients are instructed to breathe slowly and regularly (8–12 breaths per minute), inhaling through the nose and using the diaphragm in respiration. To aid clients, a pacing tape may be used. This is simply a recording of instructions to 'Breathe in' and 'Breathe out' suitably spaced to promote good breathing habits.

Client information sheet 3: **Controlling bodily feelings of anxiety**

Correct breathing

Although we tend to think that breathing comes naturally and we can all do it, there is a right and a wrong way. It is rather like standing and sitting—you can get away with bad posture for a while, but eventually it will cause you discomfort. Similarly, breathing too quickly will not seem troublesome in the short-term, but continued fast respiration causes physical discomfort which can be quite frightening. This sort of rapid breathing is a perfectly normal response to stress and is called *hyperventilation*. We all hyperventilate whenever we are tense or anxious or doing exercise. We breathe faster at these times in order to provide our muscles with oxygen to burn during activity. In this way, our body is prepared for action to relieve the stress—running away, for example.

When overbreathing becomes a habit, however, it can become a problem. Continuous overbreathing causes the oxygen levels in the blood to rise too much; at the same time, the relative carbon dioxide levels fall. This imbalance causes many unpleasant physical symptoms, such as:

- tingling face, hands, or limbs;
- muscle tremors and cramps;
- dizziness and visual problems;
- difficulty breathing;
- exhaustion and feelings of fatigue;
- chest and stomach pains...etc.

These sensations can be alarming, often causing even more anxiety and hyperventilation. You can learn to correct overbreathing and combat the symptoms for yourself by developing the habit of correct breathing. This simply means breathing gently and evenly, through your nose, filling your lungs completely. Use your lungs fully and avoid breathing from your upper chest alone. Breathing should be a smooth action, without gulping or gasping.

The breathing exercise

It is generally easier to do this exercise lying down. When you can feel the difference between shallow and deep breathing, you can try the exercise sitting or standing.

- Place one hand on your chest and one on your stomach.
- As you breathe in through your nose, allow your stomach to swell. This means that you are using your lungs fully. Try to keep the movement in your upper chest to a minimum and keep the movement gentle.
- Slowly and evenly, breathe out through your nose.
- Repeat this, while trying to get a rhythm going. You are aiming to take eight to 12 breaths a minute: breathing in and breathing out again counts as one breath.

At first you may feel that you are not getting enough air, but with practice you will find this slower rate of breathing is comfortable.

Practice

It is important to practise the exercise whenever you can as you are trying to develop a new habit, which will only come through repeated rehearsal. To help you to practise, try putting a coloured spot somewhere eye catching to remind you to use correct breathing each time you see it. A small dot of bright nail varnish should do the trick, or try a sticky spot from a memo board. You might find it useful to put the marker on your watch, as most of us look at our watches regularly throughout the day.

As your skill improves, you will find it easier to switch to correct breathing whenever you fell anxious. As with all anxiety management techniques, you will be most successful if you tackle your stress when it is at a low level.

Emergency measure

If you are feeling panicky and not confident enough to take control of your breathing pattern, use a paper bag to breathe into. Cover your nose and mouth and breathe as naturally as possible. By collecting and re-breathing your exhaled air, you can restore the oxygen/carbon dioxide balance in your bloodstream and thus control the unpleasant feelings.

Controlling anxious feelings
Under supervision, clients are requested to hyperventilate in order to induce the symptoms of anxiety. They are then told to control the symptoms through slow, nasal, diaphragmatic breathing. In this way, people learn to take control of the unpleasant feelings.

Set the homework task of regular practice of controlled breathing. For some people, it is useful to suggest that they 'cue' themselves to check their respiration regularly and, if necessary, modify this. The cue for checking respiration rate needs to be specific to the individual, and it is useful to ask each person what she or he believes would be an effective personal cue. Two commonly used reminders are the digital watch alarm which provides an auditory cue or a small coloured spot placed in a noticeable position to give a visual cue. A coloured spot might be placed on to a watch face as a reminder to check breathing rate whenever the wearer looked at the time.

Finally, invite questions to ensure that your client has a good understanding of the purpose of the exercise and its mode of application.

Dealing with problems

'*I can't breathe deeply*': It is quite common for people to have some difficulty with diaphragmatic breathing at first. You can suggest that your client tries to empty the lungs completely, blowing out vigorously. After this, people can usually inhale deeply with ease, and once this happens they tend to be more relaxed about the breathing and the whole procedure is more comfortable.

'*I don't know if I am doing this properly*': You can help your clients monitor respiration better by suggesting that they lie down for the exercise and place one or two hands on the abdomen. In this way, it is easier to feel whether the diaphragm is moving. It is possible to force diaphragmatic breathing at first by pushing out the stomach on inhalation, and this can be useful in helping clients to get the right sensation and the rhythm.

Introducing thought management

If you decide that it is necessary to teach your client how to deal with worrying thoughts, start by outlining the function of thoughts in the production and maintenance of anxiety and explain the technique of controlling the stress by tackling underlying thoughts. Use Client Information Sheet 4 to supplement your teaching.

If the identification of thoughts is difficult, ask your client to keep a thought diary as a homework task. This is not always an easy assignment, so you may need to grade it. You could simply ask for one or two entries at first, and not expect thought-challenging straight away. As your client improves at thought identification, diary keeping can become more detailed and thought-challenging can be introduced when appropriate. Always emphasize the importance of meticulous recording in the diaries.

Explain why the particular method which you have suggested will be helpful, using the handout as an aid for your client. If you introduce distraction as a coping technique, try to devise distractors which are tailored to your client's interests and life-style. For example, a woman who enjoys playing the piano might find that a certain piece of music takes her mind off worrying thoughts, or a man who grows roses for a hobby might use an image of a perfect bloom being prepared for a contest to distract him from ruminations. Reinforce suggestions which come from the client, and explain the need to practise a few distraction techniques to find out what works best and under what circumstances. Client Information Sheet 4, which discusses distraction, is on page 115.

If you intend to teach thought-challenging, you will need to go through your client's diary carefully, looking for the following common thinking errors:

- **Exaggerating**—magnifying bad points and weakness. For example, worrying about a serious reprimand at work because of a minor mistake, or panicking that a slight chest pain indicates angina, despite a good health record.

- **Catastrophizing**—anticipating that total disaster will follow a minor mishap such as predicting personal redundancy after hearing that a colleague in another department has lost her job.

- **Overgeneralizing**—translating one negative experience into a rule for life expecting *everything* to be awful, *always*, because of one bad experience; predicting a lifetime of loneliness because a relationship has just failed.

- **Ignoring the positive**—overlooking personal strengths and successful experiences, while recognizing weaknesses and failures.

Client information sheet 4: **Keeping worrying thoughts under control**

Anxiety is usually accompanied by worrying or alarming thoughts. Sometimes these are easily identified, for example, when you walk into a party, you might feel a wave of anxiety and realize that it is because you thought: 'I'll never be able to make conversation in front of all these people—I'll look silly'. At other times anxiety seems to come out of the blue and you can't think why.

Whether or not you can identify the trigger for your anxiety, a pattern of worrying thoughts and increasing anxiety can develop which will keep your tension high. For example, in the party situation, symptoms of anxiety such as blushing or not being able to speak easily would cause more worry and increase stress and social worries. A cycle of social anxiety could develop. If the situation were one where you had a slight chest pain and your thought was: 'This could be a heart attack'—your stress levels would rise, you would experience symptoms such as increased muscular tension; this would worsen your pain and your thoughts might become even more alarming: 'This *is* a heart attack!' Your anxiety would get worse, and so on. The cycle of increasing tension would develop.

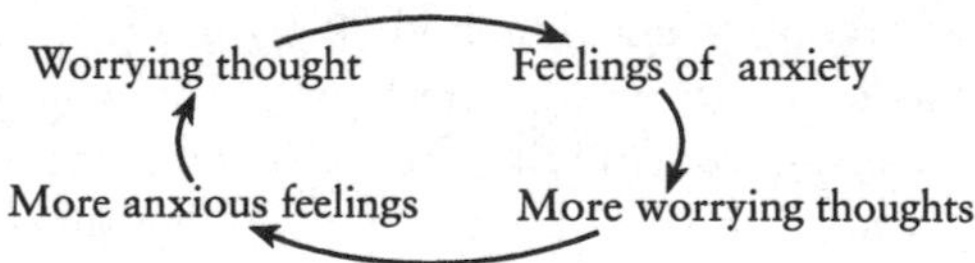

Alarming thoughts keep the anxiety going and the symptoms of anxiety maintain the alarming thoughts. It can be difficult to take your mind off unpleasant thoughts, but there are ways of overcoming this difficulty, namely: **distraction** and **challenging**.

Distraction

It is possible to concentrate on only one thing at once, so when you turn your attention to something which is neutral or pleasant, you can distract yourself from worrying thoughts. By using specific techniques of distraction, you can break the cycle of worrying thoughts and prevent your anxiety increasing. There are three basic distraction techniques which you can tailor to suit your needs. These are: physical exercise, refocusing, and mental exercise. The key to successful distraction lies in finding something which is absorbing and specific. If a distraction task is too simple or vague, it tends not to be so effective.

1. *Physical exercise*. This simply means keeping active when you are stressed. If you are physically occupied, you are less likely to be able to dwell on worrying thoughts. You could try taking exercise—which is particularly good as it helps use up the adrenalin which can otherwise make you feel tense. If, at a party, you began to feel self-conscious, you might offer to take drinks around to people to keep yourself and your mind busy. If your physical task requires mental effort, all the better because the distraction effect will be more powerful. In different situations, you will need different activities. Here are some that you might try: taking exercise out of doors, away from a stressful situation; reorganizing your garage or a room in the house if you are unable to go out; tidying your handbag or updating your diary if you are physically restricted in what you can do—in a doctor's waiting room, for example.

2. *Refocusing*. This means paying great attention to things around you, such as: counting the number of people you can see with blonde hair; looking for certain objects in a shop window; listening to others' conversations; studying the details of someone's dress or of a picture; reading the small print on tins in the supermarket. The more detailed the task the more distracting it will be.

3. *Mental exercise*. This requires you to be more creative and to use more mental effort. You might try reciting some poetry, recalling a favourite holiday trip, practising mental arithmetic, or studying someone nearby and trying to guess what they do, what interests they might have, where they are going, etc. You could try dwelling on an imaginary scene to take your mind away from worrying thoughts, and by making your scene come alive with colour and sounds and texture, you can better distract yourself.

General rules for distraction

- Choose a distraction technique which is suited to you and the situation where you need to be distracted. There is no point in dwelling on a picture of a sun-soaked beach if you hate the sea and your real love is skiing. Similarly relying on physical activity to distract you will not be helpful if your anxiety attacks are during interviews. Work out what your preferences and needs are and then tailor distraction to suit you. Try to make use of your own interests: if you are a keen gardener, you might use pruning and weeding as your physical activity; looking through the bus window at gardens and identifying plants as a refocusing exercise and holding an image of a beautiful formal garden as a mental task.

- When you have established what you need, be inventive in developing your own selection of distraction techniques, but always be specific in your choice of task and choose exercises which demand much attention.

- When you have a repertoire of distraction techniques for different occasions, practise them whenever you have the chance. In this way, when you are stressed, you can switch your thoughts to your distractor quite easily.

If your distraction technique isn't very effective, this might be because:

1. You are not practised enough. So, practise more, especially when you are not anxious.

2. The technique was not suited to the situation. Think what other strategies you have in your repertoire and give them a try.

3. You were already too stressed to manage your anxiety effectively. Try to catch your anxiety earlier next time—any coping technique will work better if you are less stressed.

A final note: Many people find distraction an invaluable anxiety management strategy. It helps to control worrying thoughts and gives a person an opportunity to think and plan more productively. However, it does not suit everyone and it can even be counter-productive if it is used as a means of avoiding difficult situations. For example, if you were anxious about speaking with people at social gatherings and you *always* handed round the drinks, then you would never face your real fear. In this instance you would need to try 'challenging' which is described in the next section.

Challenging

The technique of challenging requires you to recognize a worrying thought, ask yourself: 'Is this a realistic worry?' If it isn't a realistic concern, you need to replace it with a constructive statement. First, you must be able to identify anxious thoughts. Your best cue is feeling anxious. When you are aware of tension, ask yourself: 'What is going through my mind?' Your worries may be in the form of sentences such as : 'I am going to make a fool of myself' or 'I think I am having a heart attack', or in the form of a picture, such as a scene where you are losing control or an image of something terrible happening.

It is not always easy to recognize worrying thoughts, but it is usually a worry which triggers anxiety. If the thought is very condensed it can be difficult to realize that you have had an alarming thought. For example, if you are driving and a dog runs out in front of you, you are not aware that you think something like: 'Here is a dog running into the road. Given the speed that I am travelling and the rate at which it is crossing the road, I will hit the animal unless I do something about it'—you just use the brakes. This sort of behaviour is an automatic response to certain thoughts, anxiety can become automatic, too.

The process of challenging

There are three steps in challenging worrying thoughts: identifying them; analysing them; finding alternatives.

1. *Identifying the worrying thoughts*. When you are feeling calm, it is not always easy to identify the thoughts which trigger your anxiety. So, keeping a record of what goes through your mind during an anxious episode can be the best way of discovering the

words, images, or phrases which cause your tension. Write down whatever is in your mind when you are anxious and, with practice, this task will become easier. If you continue to find this exercise difficult, remember that timing is important: if you do not 'catch' a thought as it occurs, you can lose it. Also, try not to avoid examining what you feel and think: in the short-term, you may feel distressed by looking closely at your thoughts, but doing so will eventually enable you to take control of your worries and anxiety.

2. *Analysing thoughts*. When you keep your diary, you will need to look for some common *thinking errors* which exacerbate anxiety. These will probably fall into the categories:

- *Exaggerating*: magnifying bad points or weaknesses; for example, worrying all day about one small mistake, fearing that you will lose your job because of it. Or, panicking about a slight pain in your chest, forgetting all the signs that you are in good health.
- *Catastrophizing*: anticipating total disaster if something minor goes wrong. For example, expecting major complications when having simple, safe surgery or, the mother of the bride thinking: 'She's already three minutes late, soon everyone will leave, the wedding will be cancelled, all my efforts and money will be wasted, I will be a laughing stock,'
- *Overgeneralizing*: expecting *everything* to be awful *always* because of one bad experience. For example, predicting that you will *never* be employed again because your first job interviewer rejected you. Or, that *nobody* cares about you because one friend had rebuffed you.
- *Ignoring the positive*: overlooking personal strengths and good experiences and dwelling on the negative aspects of yourself and your life. For example, ignoring the many good grades you got at school if you have a poor mark in one test.

3. *Finding alternative ways of thinking*. There are five questions to work through to generate a more helpful way of thinking:

- *Are there reasons for my having this worrying thought*? This will help you to understand why you have the worry and make it less likely that you feel silly or embarrassed about it.

- *Are there reasons against my holding this thought*? Now you are beginning to look for evidence to undermine and weaken your worry. You might use a friend or a partner to help you come up with statements to refute your worry.
- *What is the worst thing that could happen*? Be brave and consider the worst outcome of the situation which bothers you.
- *How would I cope with this*? Now work out a plan for coping in the worst situation. If you can cope with the worst thing that could happen you can feel confident that you can manage your anxiety. Reflect on your own assets and skills and on your successful coping experiences in the past. Think about how you might change the problem situation or change how you feel about it. Also consider how others can help: what advice and support is available from family, friends or professionals? Again, you might find it helpful to get someone else's views on this.
- *What is the constructive way of viewing the situation*? Look back over the notes you have made and use them to form a new, constructive statement in response to your initial worry.

When you first start to do this exercise, you might find that it takes you some time and that you need to keep notes. As you become more practised, you will be able to work through the five questions quickly and challenging your worrying thoughts will become more automatic.

Practice

Like all other skills, challenging improves with practice. It is difficult to challenge worrying thoughts when you are distressed, so you could start by keeping a thought diary and challenging your worries after your anxiety has subsided. As you become more skilled, you can challenge your thoughts nearer the time they occur and eventually in the anxiety provoking situation itself. Do write down your challenging statements in full as they will have more impact if you spell them out and you will better develop the skill of thought challenging if you get into the habit of examining your worries thoroughly.

Eventually, the rational response to worrying thoughts can become as automatic as the anxiety response is now. However, you should expect to have 'good' days and 'bad' days as there are going to be times when you are not feeling well, or feeling tired, or just too distressed to put challenging into action in the stressful situation. At these times, try to use distraction as a way of coping with the anxiety and, when you are feeling calmer, think about the rational response to your worries and also try to understand why challenging was difficult for you on this occasion.

- **Misinterpretation**—Believing that a bodily symptom indicates a serious physical or mental condition. For example, believing that a tension headache is the result of a tumour, or that a panic attack indicates impending madness.

The next step is to help your client identify these cognitive distortions and to replace them with more rational responses. Useful questions to encourage your client to ask are: 'What evidence have I got that this terrible thing will happen?'; 'What can I do to check out my fear?'; 'What would I say reassure a friend under these circumstances?'

It is also helpful to ask: 'What's the worst thing that could happen?', followed by 'How would I deal with that?'. Considering the worst outcome can be an extremely frightening prospect for your client, especially if she or he has managed to avoid addressing it. However, with support, many can identify their terrible expectation and once this is achieved, can begin to use problem solving as a means of generating solutions. The feared outcome is never as alarming if the client is armed with coping strategies and simply doing this exercise can take the angst out of a situation.

In the early stages of thought-challenging, it is helpful to work through specific examples in the session, with the therapist modelling adaptive responses. This allows the client to rehearse under supervision and at a time when she or he is calm and best able to produce effective coping statements. The sorts of coping statement which can be useful are given below.

In preparation for stress

'I can develop a plan to deal with this—the situation is not hopeless'; 'Don't worry, it doesn't help'; 'Maybe what I think is anxiety is excitement'.

When handling a stressor

'I can meet this challenge, because I have done so in the past'; 'This feeling is not a heart attack, it is anxiety. This reminds me to use my exercise'; 'Take a slow, deep breath'.

Coping with negative feelings

'I will focus on the present, rather than thinking about difficult times in the past'; 'I expected this to happen; it is not the end of the world, now

I can use my skills to overcome these feelings'; 'I don't expect to eliminate fear, but I can keep it at a manageable level'; 'I am worried that people are laughing at me. It's no good expecting to read their minds, I can ask someone and check out my fear'; 'My mind is racing with worrying thoughts—I will think of something else'.

Reinforcement after the event

'I controlled my anxiety, and I am pleased with myself'; 'It wasn't as bad as I had expected and the control gets easier with practice'.

The principles of challenging worrying thoughts are discussed in Client Information Sheet 4, p. 115.

When clients challenge worrying thoughts, it is very important that they are not too critical of themselves. It is not helpful for them to use denigrating phrases like 'Don't be so stupid'. This would not enhance self-confidence in anyone. Each client needs to practise rational statements when calm so that they become familiar and easily employed under stress.

Finally, remember to invite questions from the client.

Dealing with problems

'*I don't have thoughts*': Many people believe that their anxiety is not mediated by worrying thoughts, although this is very unlikely. It is probable that their thoughts have become so automatic that they are only fleeting images or a trace of the original fear. The best way of identifying these cognitions is by persevering with thought diaries at the time of an anxiety attack. The most useful types of question that the therapist can ask are, 'What is going through your mind when you are anxious? What do you picture in your mind? Is there any word which triggers off anxiety?'

'*I don't believe the rational statements*': It does take some time to develop confidence in rational responses to worrying thoughts. The irrational response is often so well practised that there is quite a delay between the logical intellectual statement and emotional response. You can assure your client that the more frequent the use of rational responses, the more believable they will become.

Client information sheet 5: **Coping with a panic attack**

It is always easier to control anxiety in its early stages, and this why it is helpful to recognize the beginnings of tension. However, there may be times when you miss the early signs and you become panicky. Then it is hard to think clearly and act sensibly, so it is important to learn what to do if ever you have a panic attack. If you are well prepared, you will be able to manage your feelings.

1. Remember, *your feelings are normal and harmless.*
2. *Control frightening thoughts*: think of the situation in a more positive way.
3. *Accept what is happening to you.* If you wait, the fear will pass. If you run away, it will be more difficult to cope with the situation in the future.
4. *Practise anxiety management*: relaxation, distraction, rational thinking.
5. *Make a plan* to ease the situation. You could rest until you feel calmer or get the help of a friend, for example. Whatever you decide, carry it out in as relaxed a way as you can.

Breathing during a panic attack

When panicking, people breathe quickly and/or deeply. This is called overbreathing or hyperventilation, and it is a normal response to stress. Unfortunately, when this becomes a habit or becomes frightening in itself, overbreathing is a problem. Too much oxygen is taken into the body and very unpleasant feelings results. These sensations include tingling, aches and pains, trembling, dizziness, breathing difficulties, etc., and are so similar to the physical symptoms of anxiety that the two are often confused. The tension and anxiety which these unpleasant feelings create tend to cause more overbreathing, and a cycle is set up.

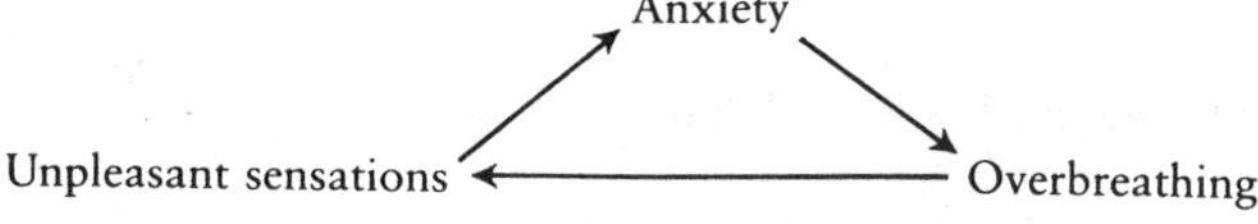

This cycle can be broken by changing your breathing pattern—even during a panic. There are two ways of doing this.

1. *Breathing into a paper bag*. Hold it tightly over your nose and mouth and breathe into the bag for several seconds. You will collect carbon dioxide in the bag. Rebreathing this air restores the oxygen/carbon dioxide balance quite quickly, and the unpleasant sensations disappear.

2. *Changing your breathing*. Slow down your breathing, try to take in air slowly and smoothly and let it out just as slowly. Breathe from your diaphragm—the muscle just below your rib-cage.

(i) First, empty your lungs, then breathe in smoothly through your nose to the slow count of four, allowing your stomach to swell.

(ii) Then, breathe out, just as smoothly, to the slow count of six. Aim to take between 8 and 12 breaths a minute, and try to get a comfortable rhythm going.

At first, you might feel that you are not getting enough air, but it is important to resist the urge to take up a quick gulp. Also, try not to breathe from your upper chest. In this way, you can restore the right oxygen/carbon dioxide balance in your body and the unpleasant sensations will disappear.

You will need to practise these breathing exercises when you are calm so that you can use the skills readily when you are anxious. You can remind yourself to practise this breathing exercise by putting a reminder where you will see it frequently. For example, a small spot of nail varnish on your watch face will remind you to check your breathing rate whenever you look at the time.

Introducing panic management

It is extremely difficult to act rationally when panicking. The client must be very familiar with coping strategies so that the techniques can be used almost automatically when she or he panics.

When discussing panic management, explain that although it is best to try to tackle anxiety in its early stages, there are ways of coping when stress builds up to a very high level. Reassure your client that panic attacks are not harmful or dangerous, and outline the physical sensations which might be expected. Also emphasize the importance of rehearsing anxiety management techniques while calm so as to be well prepared to cope with panic. Go through panic management techniques with the client, using Client Information Sheet 5 on page 124.

The handout summarizes the main points, namely that the feelings of panic are harmless and the best approach is to accept what is happening and to make a short-term coping plan which incorporates sound anxiety management skills. Portable index cards, summarizing the principles of panic management, can be a particularly helpful guide for someone who is panicking and thus not able to think, plan, and make decisions easily.

Explain the effects of overbreathing and the mechanism of anxiety maintenance through hyperventilation. If it seems useful, practise voluntary hyperventilation with your client, and teach controlled breathing.

13 *Dealing with avoidance*

As in other areas of AMT, when introducing the idea of facing the situation or the object which is feared, begin with the rationale and check your client's understanding of it. You can use Client Information Sheet 6 to help you to communicate the necessary information about the strategies which will be used, namely: graded exposure and problem solving

Graded exposure

With graded exposure, the two main points to emphasize are, the importance of taking on modest tasks at first and that the client will eventually assume the responsibility of her or his own progress. The key stages are setting targets, grading tasks, and practising.

Setting the target

Ask your client to list the situations or objects which are anxiety provoking, but which she or he expects to be able to face. You can then check that these goals are realistic. The goal, 'To improve my social life by being able to attend college parties without panicking' is realistic, while 'To find a wife and get a good job' might not be possible simply through AMT.

Each target must be very clearly defined, so that its achievement is unambiguous. 'Driving alone' is too vague; 'Driving on my own, to Crewe, on a weekday and parking in the multi-storey car park' is better. Next, arrange the targets in order of difficulty and select the easiest item as the first goal to aim for. It is possible to start with a more difficult one if this is more urgent, although success may then not be achieved so quickly.

In the early stages of therapy, it is wise not to tackle more than one goal at a time. You might find that you have to restrain an overenthusiastic client in order to prevent that person from attempting too many

Client information sheet 6: **Facing the fear**

Facing fear: graded practice

There are many different fears or phobias: fears of heights, travelling, animals, busy places, etc.; the list is endless. No matter what you fear, you can learn to control the anxiety and overcome your phobia.

First you must understand *your* fear: you need to know exactly what frightens *you*. For example, you might say that you are afraid of spiders but this could mean quite different things for different people. One person might be able to tolerate a medium size spider at the other side of the room, and only become frightened if that spider moved nearer. Another person may become panicky just looking at a picture of a small spider. Someone with a spider phobia needs to ask: What size of spider makes me feel anxious? How near can I tolerate the spider? Does it make a difference where I am, or what time of day it is? Does it make a difference if I am with someone?

Another example could be a fear of shopping. This is a rather vague description of a phobia and, if you have this type of fear you need to ask yourself: Which shops make me particularly anxious? What time of the day is worse or better for me? What makes it easier or harder for me to cope?

By asking yourself these sorts of questions for each of your fears, you will be able to describe your problem in sufficient detail for you to use the techniques of *graded practice*. You may have more than one specific fear, if so, do this exercise for each of your fears.

Avoidance

People often avoid things or situations which frighten them, but by avoiding, a person never gets the chance to discover whether or not that fear is realistic and never gets the opportunity to learn to deal with the fear and overcome it. In fact, the more someone avoids, the harder it becomes to face up to a source of anxiety. Therefore it is important to face one's fear.

Facing the fear one step at a time

Tackling your fear one step at a time is known as *graded practice*. This approach helps you to overcome your fear by providing the opportunity to learn that certain situations or objects are not really dangerous or frightening. Practising in the situation which makes you feel uncomfortable or frightened actually reduces anxiety—as long as the practice tasks are organized in the right way.

Although the notion of facing your fear might seem alarming, you can learn to do it gradually, so that you never need feel very afraid when carrying out graded practice. First, you can attempt something relatively easy and then move on to more challenging situations at your own pace. In this way, you will build up your confidence again. There are three stages in graded practice:

1. Setting targets.
2. Grading tasks.
3. Practising.

Setting targets

Take the list of the situations which you avoid or which make you very anxious arrange your fears in order of difficulty. These are your *targets*. You might have a list like:

Most difficult:

1. Shopping in the hypermarket, alone, on Friday evening, when it is most busy.
2. Taking the bus from home into town (4 miles), alone, in the morning when it's crowded.
3. Using the lift at work (from the bottom floor to level seven) when there is nobody around.

Least difficult:

4. Sitting in the centre of the row in a cinema or theatre, with my partner.

When you have your targets ranked according to difficulty, select the easiest one to start with. If one of the targets is particularly urgent, you might choose to begin with that one instead. At this stage, you should only tackle one at a time. You will work your way to achieving this target in safe, graded steps.

Grading the tasks

You now need to plan a series of small, specific tasks of increasing difficulty, which culminate in your target. The first task has to be achievable, so ask yourself: 'Can I imagine myself doing this with a bit of effort?' If you answer 'No,' then make the task easier. It is essential that you do not take risks: the aim of graded practice is to build on a series of successes, so you have to plan for success. Each task has to be described in detail, for example:

TARGET: Shopping in the hypermarket, alone, on Friday evening.

TASKS:

1. Shopping in the comer shop, with my friend, on Thursday afternoon, when it is quiet. Buying just one item, which I can pick up easily and take to the shopkeeper. I will have the correct change in my hand.
2. Ditto, buying three items which I can pick up easily and paying with a note so that I have to wait for the change.
3. Ditto, buying at least ten items from a shopping list and paying with a note.

..., etc.

This is the starting point for graded practice, the tasks could develop in various ways before the target is reached. For example, starting to shop alone and building on that, or beginning by taking on larger shops, or starting shopping at busier times. Only try to change one aspect of a task at a time and accommodate practical constraints. For example, if a friend were only available for a short time, it would be important to become independent of her before changing the task to a busier time or a larger shop.

In summary, the rest of the graded practice might look like this:

4. Using the local shop, at a quiet time on my own.
5. Using the shop, alone, at a medium- busy time.

6. Using the shop, alone, at the busiest time.
7. Using a mini-market, alone, at a quiet time.
8. Using a mini-market, alone, at a busy time.
9. Using the supermarket, alone, at a quiet time.
10. Using the supermarket, alone, at a busy time.
11. Using the hypermarket, alone, at a quiet time.
12. Using the hypermarket, alone, at a busy time.

Practising

Practise each step, using your coping skills, until you can manage it without difficulty. Then, and only then, move on to the next task. Don't be put off by some feelings of anxiety—this is only natural. Remember that you are learning to master anxiety instead of avoiding it. To be helpful, practice has to be:

- *regular* and frequent enough for the benefits not to be lost;
- *rewarding*—recognize your achievements and learn to praise yourself.
- *repeated* until the anxiety is no longer there;

If you find that a task is too difficult, don't give up or feel that you have failed. Instead, look for ways of making the task easier—perhaps as two or three smaller steps. Expect set-backs from time to time and when this happens, think about your task. Did you overestimate what you could do and make the task too difficult? Did you practise when you were feeling unwell or tired? Did you have other things on your mind so that you could not put enough effort into your practice? If you keep a record of your practice, you can more easily work out why you have difficulties on certain days. Also, by keeping a dairy you have a long-term record of your progress.

Don't forget to give yourself praise for your achievements, no matter how small. Try not to downgrade your successes and try not to criticize yourself: encouragement works better. In this way, you will manage to reach your goals and face your fears with confidence.

Facing the fear: problem solving and decision making

Graded practice is the best way of facing your fear if you have the time to organize a programme for yourself, but sometimes this isn't possible because a stressful event is imminent and you don't have time to follow a step by step approach. You might be confronted by a wholly unexpected event, or you may have to tackle something that you have ignored and now find that you have little time to prepare for it. Whatever the situation, being faced with an immediate problem often triggers panic and it becomes even more difficult to plan how to cope.

There are six steps which you can take to make your task easier.

1. *Define the problem.* Be specific about the task ahead and try not to confuse several tasks. Where possible, distinguish the different aspects of your problem and separate it into a collection of more manageable tasks, then make a plan for each. For each task ask: What is going to happen? When will this happen? Who is involved? Only work on one task at a time. At the end of this stage, you should be able to say what your goal is, in very specific terms.

2. *List solutions.* Think of as many ways of dealing with the problem as you can. Write them all out, no matter how trivial or outrageous they might seem. At this stage, you are aiming to generate a wide range of possible courses of action. The more you come up with the better. It might be helpful to put yourself in someone else's shoes and consider how that person might respond if asked to deal with your problem.

3. *Evaluate the pros and cons of each solution.* Consider each action plan and decide which will have to be rejected because of unsuitability. Next, reflect on the remainder and rank order the solutions from least to most useful for you at this time. Take your first choice solution.

4. *Plan*: In very specific and concrete terms, decide how you are going to implement your chosen solution. Be sure to answer: What will be done? How will it be done? When will it be done? Who is involved? Where will it take place? What is my contingency plan?

A contingency plan is a back-up plan which you can put into operation if your task is more difficult than you anticipated or something unexpected turns up and prevents you from carrying through your original course of action. For example, you might carry the telephone number of a friend whom you can ring to collect you from a wedding or whom you can talk to if you get nervous just before an interview.

Where possible, rehearse either in imagination or with someone who could role play with you. Also, scan all your solutions to see if you might profitably combine them. For example, you might find that 'Asking my friend to rehearse with me what I might say'; links very well with, 'Preparing myself by relaxing before I see my boss.'

5. *Action*. Try out your solution.

6. *Evaluate yourself.* If your solution works and is sufficient, congratulate yourself and remember this successful experience for the future. If your solution does not solve your problem, try to understand why it went wrong—perhaps you were over-ambitious, perhaps you were not feeling strong that day, perhaps you misjudged someone else's response to you. Whatever conclusion you reach, remember that *you did not fail*. Expect some disappointments but commend yourself for having tried. Learn as much as you can from the experience and go back to your solution list and select the next one.

You can continue to return to your list of solutions as often as you need to. The more solutions you are able to generate, the greater will be your store of options.

Problem solving is a useful technique when prompt action is necessary. However, it is always better to plan well in advance when you are able to do so. Try not to put off thinking about a difficult task until the last moment.

targets too soon. Only attempt to achieve targets which the client ***wants*** to tackle. An ambivalent client will not be well motivated to take on a challenge that is not really necessary. For example, your client might be fearful of using public transport but, if she never needs to use it, she is unlikely to want to go through the trauma of overcoming her fear.

Grading the target

Plan a series of small, specific tasks of increasing difficulty, which culminate in the target. The first task in this hierarchy must be achievable, so ask your client, 'What are you pretty sure you could manage with a little effort?' At this stage, it is essential that you do not take risks: the aim of graded exposure is to build on a series of successes, so you have to plan for success.

Each task should be clearly described (who, where, what, when) so that your client knows exactly what is to be carried out and be certain when this has been achieved. Uncertainty promotes anxiety and an ambiguous achievement is often dismissed by the client.

In the early stages of graded exposure, take only one task at a time. Later, as your clients become more proficient at this technique, other tasks can be attempted at the same time. As clients become more experienced, they can take on the role of planner.

Practising

Once you and your client have established one or more hierarchies, the exposure work begins. As has already been discussed, this can take place in the session, in imagination, or in the actual setting. The last is the most common setting and the exposure is carried out in the form of homework assignments.

When you follow an exposure programme, prepare the client for the anxious feelings which are likely to be experienced and remind him or her that the goal is to master anxiety, not to eliminate it. Begin with the first task in the hierarchy and when this has been done more than once without difficulty, move on to the next step. Make sure that your client appreciates that, to be effective, practice must be frequent and regular and at least daily, if possible. The salient points of graded practice are shown in part 1 of Client Information Sheet 6 on page 127.

It is helpful if the client keeps a record of achievement as an indicator of progress. This need comprise only the task performed and an associated anxiety rating.

Prepare people for the occasional set-back as this is bound to occur from time to time and is part of normal progress. Also, review progress regularly, collecting feedback from record sheets and verbal report. Reinforce your client's achievements, and use the feedback to modify the current plan if this is necessary, and to prepare future programmes.

Problem solving

When your client has to face a difficult situation with little time for graded exposure, or when a task does not lend itself to planned desensitization, then you can introduce problem solving. This technique encourages the client to stand back from the problem and then generate and evaluate as many solutions as possible. The steps involved can be seen in part 2 of Client Information Sheet 6 on page 127.

One of the great advantages of the problem-solving approach is that it provides a well defined series of steps that the client can turn to when in crisis. Decision making can be kept to a minimum at a time when it is likely to be impaired; the client simply slips into the routine.

With problem solving, the production of many solutions is crucial, but clients are often inhibited about making suggestions which they do not think correct or good enough. It can be helpful, therefore, if the therapist and client engage in the task together and the therapist illustrates how to generate solutions which are not vetted and may even be rather odd.

Dealing with problems

'I have failed': Explain that not completing a task does not indicate failure, but often results from over-optimistic planning. The positive aspect of set-backs is that you and your clients can learn more about personal limitations and plan more realistically next time. It might be helpful if you predict that people will have 'good' and 'bad' days, and encourage acceptance of this. Set-backs and lapses are bound to occur and it should be emphasized that these are not the same as failures and relapses and that even those events which might be construed as 'failures' provide the opportunity for learning. Also, warn your clients that performance can be impaired through illness, fatigue, or stress, and emphasize that this reflects no fault in the person.

Downgrading success: This is a common response to success, and one which undermines confidence and demoralizes the client. The aim of graded practice is to develop a sense of self-efficacy and build self-confidence, so you need to stress the importance of acknowledging all achievements, no matter how small. You can enhance this by recognizing and reinforcing successes and also by ensuring that tasks are very concrete and observable, thus avoiding the ambiguity which frequently results in downgrading.

Management plans: case examples

A case of generalized anxiety: Mrs Green

Mrs Green agreed with the formulation of her problem which her GP had presented. This then formed the basis of her treatment plan. Given her particular resources, namely a friend who was willing to be involved in therapy and no financial restrictions, they agreed an approach which would involve:

- relaxation training to deal with the physical symptoms;
- distraction to help her to combat the worrying thoughts;
- graded exposure to public transport to help her overcome avoidance

The GP acted as therapist, seeing Mrs Green weekly for a month, then at 2-weekly intervals over the next month. At first they agreed on five therapy sessions, but reviewed this in session five and decided that six were necessary. They also agreed that Mrs Green should contact the GP after 3 months (unless she needed to consult before) to discuss her progress.

Relaxation training

At this particular practice, an occupational therapist (OT) ran a 3-week course in relaxation training. She held two group sessions per week, teaching PMR skills followed by instruction in applying these in anxiety-provoking situations. The OT also taught controlled breathing. Mrs Green was immediately able to join a group and was encouraged to monitor her progress over the 3 weeks. By the end of this period, she began to use her unpleasant physical sensations as a cue to relax. As she became more efficient at controlling the symptoms of tension, her general anxiety diminished.

Distraction

The GP presented the rationale for distraction and Mrs Green went away to experiment with different techniques and subjects in order to discover for herself what worked best for her. After a week, Mrs Green had found that reciting short passages of scripture gave her pleasure and comfort and was thus distracting for her. She began to use distraction when she was aware of worrying thoughts racing through her mind. She found distraction effective, particularly during church services when she had to stand for some time. She kept a diary so that she might properly evaluate the efficacy of this strategy.

Graded exposure

Within a month, Mrs Green felt confident that she could control the bodily symptoms and thoughts associated with anxiety when she was at home. She and the GP collaborated in devising this graded hierarchy of five steps to achieve her goal of 'travelling to Birmingham, using a bus and the train, by myself, on a weekday, to see my son'.

Step 1: Walking to the village green with a friend.

Step 2: Walking to the village green and catching the bus to the station (three stops), with her friend.

Step 3: Step 1 and 2, alone.

Step 4: Meeting her friend at the station and taking a short train journey (20 minutes) to an exhibition.

Step 5: Taking the train to see her son (90-minute journey), alone but being met from the train by him.

To increase the likelihood of success, each step was made pleasurable and each had been negotiated for safety. In practice, she achieved her goal in six steps, as the transition from step 4 to step 5 was too great, and she first made the 90-minute journey with her son who was travelling home after visiting his mother.

A case of simple phobia: Mrs Smith

Having presented an acceptable formulation to Mrs Smith, the health visitor was able to make some suggestions for intervention. She said that she would first discuss this with the primary care team, but that she expected that Mrs Smith could learn to manage her problem in two stages:

1. Relaxation training to help her combat the physical symptoms, and the alarming imagery.
2. Graded exposure to wasps.

The health visitor recognized that any intervention would have to be immediate, before the wasp season ended, and that it would probably have to take place in Mrs Smith's home as she would find it very difficult to get someone to look after her children on a regular basis so that she could attend a clinic.

The health visitor discussed Mrs Smith's difficulties with the primary care team, and it was agreed that it would be reasonable in this case for her to take on the role of therapist. The approach which the health visitor then put to Mrs Smith was a programme of desensitization which would involve her learning brief relaxation and imagery control, coupled with graded practice. Therapy took place in Mrs Smith's home, and took five sessions to complete.

Initially, Mrs Smith could not even think about constructing a graded hierarchy of exposure without becoming panicky. The health visitor therefore first introduced relaxation, then helped Mrs Smith apply this while thinking of difficult situations.

Brief relaxation

Using the client instruction sheets as an aid, the health visitor explained the rationale behind relaxation training and taught Mrs Smith the simple relaxation routine. In this case, the mental device used was the word 'calm', as a soothing mental picture would interfere with the planned graded exposure in imagination. Mrs Smith agreed to practice the routine twice a day, when she knew that she would have an uninterrupted quarter of an hour. She rated her anxiety level before and after the exercise, using a simple five-point scale. After the first week, it was clear that she was reliably reducing her tension levels through relaxation.

Graded exposure: in imagination

The next step was to help Mrs Smith learn to tolerate the thought of wasps, prior to working with a live insect. She and the health visitor negotiated a graded exposure plan which would be carried out in imagination, the first step being one which Mrs Smith felt confident about achieving.

Goal 'To imagine holding a jar, containing a live wasp which crawls out and walks over Mrs Smith's hand'.

Step 1: Imagining a wasp in the next room and bringing anxiety ratings down to 1, by using relaxation skills and the word 'calm'.

Step 2: Imagining a wasp in a jar 12, feet away.

Step 3: Ditto with the wasp 8 feet away.

Step 4: Ditto with the wasp 4 feet away.

Step 5: Ditto with the wasp 2 feet away.

Step 6: Ditto with the wasp in a jar next to Mrs Smith.

Step 7: Ditto with Mrs Smith holding a jar with a dead wasp in it.

Step 8: Ditto with a live wasp in the jar.

Step 9: Imagining the wasp now crawling out over her gloved hand.

Step 10: Imagining the wasp crawling out over her bare hand.

The health visitor was present during this phase of desensitization. Mrs Smith was very efficient at imagining the wasp, and it took only two sessions for her to reach step 10. Mrs Smith then felt ready to progress to exposure *in vivo*.

Graded exposure in vivo

Mrs Smith worked out this programme for herself.

Goal 'To shop at the local greengrocer's on a warm summer's day'.

Step 1: Dead wasp in jar next to Mrs Smith.

Step 2: Holding jar containing dead wasp.

Step 3: Live wasp in jar next to Mrs Smith.

Step 4: Holding jar containing live wasp.

Step 5: Opening kitchen and living-room windows for 30 minutes.

Step 6: Opening the windows from noon until 5 p.m.

Step 7: Sitting in the garden for 30 minutes.

Step 8: Sitting in the garden from noon until 5 p.m.

Step 9: Shopping at the greengrocer's on a dull day.

Step 10: Shopping at the greengrocer's on a sunny day.

Following the exposure in imagination, she was able to progress to the top of her hierarchy in 3 weeks. Steps 1–3 were carried out with the health visitor present. She then continued by herself, omitting step 9 because her confidence had improved sufficiently to make this step redundant.

A case of panic attack: Mr Peters

Once they had agreed on the formulation of the problem, Mr Peters and his doctor began to devise a treatment plan based on it. The particular resources which were pertinent in Mr Peter's case were: a supportive wife who could be involved in the treatment, and freedom to organize his own work-load and travel commitments. The GP suggested that therapy would focus on helping Mr Peters develop techniques for controlling the physical and the cognitive symptoms of panic, which he would gradually be encouraged to use while driving. She gave Mr Peters information sheets about panic attack and controlling worrying thoughts and also suggested that he keep a thought diary in the car to record exactly what went through his mind as near to the time of the attack as possible.

With Mr Peters's agreement, his GP handed over responsibility for his therapy to the practice nurse, who had a particular interest and training in stress management. He met Mr Peters, at the surgery, over five treatment sessions.

In their first session together they discussed the formulation to establish that they had a shared concept of the problem, and then went on to review the thought diary. They identified two themes in his thinking. The first was 'helplessness': 'What can I do?; I can't cope; I am going to pass out; I am going to die'. The second theme was 'escape': 'Where can I pull off the road; I am only one mile from a hospital—I must get there; If I can survive for a few minutes longer, I will get home'. They negotiated a three-stage approach: developing a sense a mastery over the physical symptoms, developing coping statements which focused on good health rather than escape, and planned practice.

Developing a sense of mastery

In this first session, the practice nurse decided to carry out a voluntary hyperventilation exercise in order to establish if Mr Peters' symptoms were the result of overbreathing. With a paper bag nearby, the nurse instructed Mr Peters to breathe deeply and quickly through his mouth. Within a minute, Mr Peters was pale, shaking, and terrified that he was about to have a heart attack. This experience persuaded both client and therapist that hyperventilation played a part in the problem and they discussed the physiological basis of Mr Peters's frightening physical sensations. The nurse then taught him the technique of controlled breathing, and in the safety of the surgery, Mr Peters was able to induce and control the physical symptoms of overbreathing. His homework, for the first week, was to practise controlled breathing using a small coloured spot on his watch face as a cue to rehearse. He quickly became proficient in controlling minor stress episodes at home and at work.

Developing useful coping statements

Once Mr Peters became aware of the role of his worrying thoughts in the maintenance of his anxiety, he attempted to generate rational coping statements. However, his diaries showed that he was unable to do this when he panicked. Therefore, in the next session when he was relaxed and able to think logically, he and the practice nurse worked out a set of rational responses to his catastrophic thoughts. He was then able to rehearse these statements when he was relaxed and would later use them *in situ*. For example:

Automatic thought: This is a heart attack. I will pass out at the wheel and cause a crash.

Response: No, these are the physical symptoms of anxiety.

Automatic thought: This is a heart attack, like the one which killed my father.

Response: My father was overweight and a very heavy smoker and therefore at much greater a risk of physical illness than I am. In fact, I know that I am healthy because of the results of my medical examinations.

Mr Peters first reproduced these statements on small index cards, and took them home to read through every day for a week. By the end of the week, he was able to reduce them to a set of three key words, which reminded him of the entire statement.

Planned practice

So far, it had been possible for Mr Peters to organize his work so that he did not have to travel alone in the car. Now that he had developed skills in managing the physical and psychological symptoms of stress, he felt ready to work towards driving independently again. First, he read the handout on graded practice, then he and the practice nurse worked out a series of steps for him to work through. With his set of 'coping words' fixed inside his windscreen so that they did not obscure his vision, but placed so that he could read them as a quick glance, he began his graded exposure.

Goal

'To drive to Paris, staying overnight in a hotel'

Step 1: Driving into the village on Sunday, Wednesday, and Saturday to watch his son play football. (He had made this journey with his wife a few times, and felt ready to tackle it alone.)

Step 2: Driving into the village, with his wife, on a weekday to pick up some shopping.

Step 3: The same journey, alone.

Step 4: Driving to his office, 5 miles away, using the motorway.

Step 5: Short business journey to a large town, alone, in the week.

Step 6: Longer business journey to London, alone, on a weekday.

Step 7: Ditto, staying overnight in a hotel in London.

Step 8: Business trip to Paris: driving the distance and staying overnight in a hotel.

Mr Peters was keen to become as independent as possible as quickly as possible, and wanted to carry out his graded practice without the support of the practice nurse. As there was a danger of Mr Peters attempting to do too much and risking a set-back, the practice nurse negotiated that they would meet for two more sessions to ensure that Mr Peters was pacing himself safely. They also agreed to meet for a review session 3 months later.

A case of obsessional–compulsive behaviour: Mr Oldham

Mr and Mrs Oldham and the CPN negotiated a plan for therapy which was based on the formulation of Mr Oldham's problem. It incorporated the following points:

- developing a better understanding of obsessional–compulsive behaviour;
- learning techniques for coping with the associated physical and cognitive symptoms;
- using adaptive coping strategies in order to resist the impulse to check.

The CPN gave the couple the client information sheets which dealt with the development of problem anxiety, coping with the physical symptoms of anxiety, and managing worrying thoughts. These were discussed in their first treatment session, and the CPN took the opportunity to praise Mrs Oldham for not reinforcing her husband's avoidance, and to look at how she might take a more active role in his recovery.

This first session was held in the Oldham's home and involved two aspects of treatment.

Relaxation training with distraction

It was explained to Mr Oldham that in order to break the vicious cycle of checking and worrying, he would need to be able to overcome the physical tension and worrying thoughts which compelled him to check. To achieve this, the CPN taught him the shortened progressive relaxation technique, and gave him a tape of the instructions to use as a guide when he practised independently. To give him encouragement to practise, Mrs Oldham volunteered to join him in the exercises. Before and after each exercise, he was asked to rate his tension levels on a simple five-point scale, where a rating of 'one' indicated a very relaxed state. He was able to practise three times a day and, within a week, could reliably achieve a rating of one.

At the end of the exercise, it was suggested that Mr Oldham should focus on a relaxing image, which would further deepen his relaxation and would distract his thoughts from his worries. He practised with a few images, and discovered that 'reading' a favourite piece of music in his mind was the most distracting and pleasurable thing for him. Again, by the end of the first week, he was able to picture a manuscript of music at the end of his relaxation exercise, and respond to it. Linking the imagery with the relaxation exercise strengthened the association between the music and a feeling of calm. Soon, simply imagining the manuscript calmed him.

Over the next two sessions, the CPN instructed the Oldhams how to reduce the length of the exercise and, by practising between sessions, they developed the ability to relax to cue.

Response prevention

Over the first week, Mr Oldham had simply recorded how often he felt the compulsion to check something (at home and at work), how frequently he had resisted the impulse, and an indication of when this happened and what was the focus of concern. This served as a baseline record of his behaviour, so that they could evaluate the effect of introducing response prevention. This approach was introduced in the second session, which was also carried out in the Oldham's home, with Mrs Oldham present. The CPN asked

Mr Oldham if there was anything which he felt compelled to check at that moment. Mr Oldham replied that he had a slight urge to go into the kitchen to make sure that the gas oven was properly turned off. The CPN instructed him to close his eyes, focus on this worry, and to raise his hand when he felt that he could hardly resist checking. Mr Oldham complied, and at the moment the raised his hand, the CPN told him to think of his relaxing mental image, and to drop his hand only when the urge to check had gone. After several trials, Mr Oldham was able to elicit his worrying thought and then control the associated anxiety.

With the CPN they then studied the recording Mr Oldham had made over the previous week and derived a list of 'vulnerable times and situations', and they ranked these according to degree of vulnerability. For example, Mr Oldham always had very powerful urges to return to the office safe and check that it was locked, and he never resisted this compulsion. In contrast, he had fleeting urges to check that the car doors were locked after the garage doors had been secured, and he rarely gave into these. He now had a graded hierarchy to work through in his imagination. His homework for that week was to imagine situations and to control his impulse to check, as he had done in the practice session. As with all graded exposure plans, he began with the easiest situation, and only progressed up the list when he felt confident that he could tackle the next step. He continued to keep his record of checking impulses and behaviours, and was supported by his wife, who encouraged him to practise his coping skills at least once everyday.

By the end of a week, he had reached the top of his hierarchy. Concordantly, he had found that he was less likely to give into impulses which occurred spontaneously. This was reflected in his recordings. The CPN then suggested that he began to resist the checking behaviour at home by using his relaxation and distraction techniques. They agreed that the CPN should call again in 4 weeks' time to check on his progress. Over the month, he became proficient at resisting the impulse to check, and Mrs Oldham was always prepared to reinforce his achievements. Over the next month he transferred these skills to the office. This turned out to be easier than Mr Oldham had expected. He discovered that many of his office checking behaviours had disappeared as he gained mastery over checking at home, and he was now so well rehearsed in applying relaxation and distraction, that it came to him quite easily despite his not having the active support of his wife. His record of unwanted behaviours showed a steady decline in checking over 2 weeks, and he did not have any entries for the last fortnight.

A case of PTSD: Mr Thomas

When she shared the formulation, the counsellor also explained, to Mr Thomas, the psychological sequelae of trauma. He was much relieved to discover that the flashbacks, in particular, were quite usual in PTSD. He agreed that the maintaining cycles of his current difficulties were: the recurring images of the accident, depressed mood, and avoidance. He felt, however, that he could not begin to face his fears of driving while he was feeling so miserable and while he experienced flashbacks. Therefore, the provisional plan was as follows:

- distraction and image restructuring to help him combat flashbacks;
- reassessment by the GP to discuss the usefulness of antidepressants;
- graded exposure to driving and allowing his son to be driven.

The counsellor saw Mr Thomas twice weekly for half-hour sessions for the first fortnight and then once a week until the exposure programme was under way. The GP did feel that antidepressant medication was appropriate and within 3 weeks of taking it, Mr Thomas was less pessimistic and more physically and psychologically motivated.

Distraction

The rationale of distraction appealed to Mr Thomas and he had devised several techniques to help him. His 'physical' distraction strategy was simply running his tongue around his mouth and counting his teeth, while his refocusing task was listening to a particularly compelling piece of jazz. Both of these could be safely carried out in the car.

Image restructuring

The restructuring work was begun in sessions after Mr Thomas had learnt how to relax. In this state, he was asked to focus on his flashback, with a view to changing the ending when his anxiety levels rose. As he described the content of his flashback, his anxiety suddenly increased at the moment of recalling the red light changing to amber. He was then urged to imagine a non-stressful sequel and he was able to picture his responding to the green light and moving off safely.

This restructured image was rehearsed as an assignment and his anxiety levels, in response to the image of changing lights, diminished. Mr. Thomas' description of this process was 'rescripting', which he associated it with his line of work which gave him confidence in the strategy.

Next, he continued the flashback, past the point of the lights changing and his anxiety shot up at the moment of impact with the lorry. Mr Thomas then devised a new image of the lorry rebounding from his car, leaving it unharmed. Again, the new scenario was practised until he was able to follow through with the flashback to the point when he saw the cyclist, trapped and bleeding. This was the most difficult aspect of the flashback to 're-script', and at first he could not respond to the counsellor's question: 'What would you want to happen instead'. Eventually he replied that he wanted the cyclist to open her eyes and tell him that she would be all right and that she did not blame him. He then incorporated this into his latest image and found that it brought down his stress to a bearable level. After practising this image for some time, he found that he was now able to tolerate his original memory and felt confident that he could curtail it if he needed to.

Rational self-talk

A further cognitive obstacle, in Mr Thomas' case, was his belief that: 'I am a disappointment, no one is going to want to bother with me'. The counsellor felt that this was such a deep rooted belief that it would be better dealt with by a cognitive therapist. He had also been troubled by a further thought that: 'I'll never be free of this problem'. This cognition, however, had diminished as he gained more mastery over the flashback.

Graded exposure

Once Mr Thomas was confident that he could control the flashbacks and was feeling more able to challenge his negative thinking, he was able to contemplate a programme of planned exposure. He was clear that his goal was to pick up his son from school and he thought that his starting point would have to be simply sitting in the car with Robert. His hierarchy comprised the following steps:

Step 1: Sitting in the car in our own drive, with Robert in the child seat next to me.

Step 2: Starting up the car and driving to the end of our drive.

Step 3: Ditto, then turning left into the road and going round the block.

Step 4: Ditto, but taking a right turn.

Step 5: Driving in the vicinity of the school, with Robert, on a Sunday.

Step 6: Driving to the school, past the accident spot, with Robert, on a Sunday.

Step 7: Driving to the school to pick up Robert, on a weekday.

In practice, steps 5–7 had to be modified to, first, involve Mrs Thomas as the transitions were too difficult for Mr Thomas to take on alone. Mr Thomas also discovered that he needed to practise each step several times in order to gain his confidence and he had to repeat steps 5 and 6 in the evenings when the traffic was quiet. He kept a progress diary throughout the treatment phase.

A case of executive stress: Dr Evans

Once Dr Evans had agreed to a trial of ten 20-minute sessions, the first step, in her treatment programme, was diary keeping. The GP drew up one which required Dr Evans to jot down what she was doing each hour of the day: his rationale was that they needed to know more about the correlates of performance. She then gave herself a performance rating each hour: a rating of 5 indicated a good performance, while I meant that she had done badly. The GP explained that, if Dr Evans was amenable, they would move on to relaxation training to help her combat the unpleasant physiological symptoms of stress and they would discuss social changes which she might introduce to reduce her tension levels. Dr Evans said that this was all very well but she had a conference looming—what was the GP going to do about her inability to represent the company? Her doctor explained that, once Dr Evans had acquired some sound stress management strategies, she could start planning for the conference and that she would be encouraged to do this in a systematic way which would help her regain her old confidence.

Self-monitoring

The first week of diary keeping was productive: the self-monitoring sheets showed that the more Dr Evans squeezed into the day, the poorer was her performance; the later she worked at night, the less well she did the next day and so on. She began to accept that pushing herself was counter-productive and agreed to experiment with taking more breaks during the day.

Dr Evans was not good at identifying 'stress' because she labelled it excitement. To help her develop the skill of stress awareness, so that she might introduce stress management before her tension levels became a problem, her GP asked her to rate 'physical discomfort' every hour. It was quite easy to incorporate this into her original diary. This helped Dr Evans develop the habit of taking a brief break to check her tension levels instead of working non-stop because of the thrill she got from her job. Within a week or two, she was able to discriminate between 'safe' stress levels and 'warning signs'.

Relaxation training with controlled breathing

Her GP now introduced relaxation training and controlled breathing. He began with a brief exercise as Dr Evans was not hopeful that she would find half an hour a day to practise lengthy PMR exercises. The agreement was that she would carry out a 5- or 10-minute exercise whenever she took a break for coffee or lunch. Sometimes this meant doing the exercise in a lay-by, if she was travelling, but it was possible to incorporate brief relaxation into her daily routine. This brief exercise was enhanced by the introduction of a relaxing image. For Dr Evans, this was sliding down into a comfortable seat in a first class airline compartment, knowing that the phone could not ring, none of her staff could disturb her, and that the next few hours were hers alone.

Social changes

Within 3 weeks, she found that she was able to take things easier at work without the quality of her work suffering. In fact, her performance ratings had improved and, as she relaxed more, her period pains seemed more bearable. However, she complained that she 'missed the adrenalin' at work. She and the GP discussed the pros and cons of increasing stress at work and Dr Evans decided against it. Instead, she developed 'exciting' recreations. The twins had begged her to take them to the local 'Laser Quest' and she finally gave in, only to find that she enjoyed it. She then built on this discovery by joining sailing club which gave her adult company, competition, and excitement. Her husband was also keen and the two of them developed their social life for the first time since their marriage.

Graded practice

By now, she accepted that her work and well-being benefited from stress management, her confidence had returned but she was still apprehensive about representing her company in Paris. There were 6 weeks to go and this gave her time to embark on a programme of graded practice.

Step 1: The first step was drafting her presentation.

Step 2: The second was discussing it with her husband in an informal way.

Step 3: The third step was a strict rehearsal with only her husband present.

Step 4: After this, she felt able to present to her department and the feedback was so positive that she felt confident in committing herself to the Paris conference.

Before the presentation in Paris, she made sure that there would be the opportunity to run through the talk with her boss and gain reassurance that her performance was acceptable.

14 *Self-management and ending therapy*

You can only establish whether or not your client is developing the skills of self-management by reviewing progress regularly. Look for an understanding of the problem's maintaining factors and personal vulnerability factors, an ability to apply psychological coping techniques in response to difficulties and an ability to problem solve and plan. When all these criteria are met, you can consider ending AMT.

If you decide that it is time to finish the therapy, give advance warning of the termination date. Your client may need time to adjust to the idea that support will be withdrawn. Discuss self-management with your client and work out a personal blueprint by anticipating future difficulties and devising management plans. The important points to remember when coping independently are summarized in Client Information Sheet 7 on the following page.

Elicit questions from your client and try to identify any worries. It is best not to leave this until the very last session, when people are reluctant to express doubts and confront new issues. Give information and advice which will help your particular client cope in the long term. For example, suggest relevant literature, give lists of suitable support groups, recommend further therapies or activities. You can find a short list of useful books and addresses for your client in Appendix 8.

Emphasize the client's need to modify her or his life-style by keeping active, incorporating pleasurable activities into the daily routine, carrying out relaxation exercises regularly and keeping a diary of achievements. Benefit is also derived from modifying outlook, that is, putting the client's needs first, giving credit for successes of any magnitude, rational thinking in the face of stress, problem solving and planning when faced with a difficulty.

Your client may become apprehensive about the termination of therapy. When this is the case, reassure the individual that you can only consider termination because of your confidence in her or his ability to cope, and that support will continue to be available in an emergency. In the final session, make a specific follow-up appointment in order to review progress.

Client information sheet 7: **Long-term coping with anxiety**

You have now acquired the skills to deal with your present problems but you will have to continue to work to maintain your achievements and cope with problem anxiety for the rest of your life. The most effective way of doing this is to keep on practising.

Stress-proofing yourself

You can further 'stress-proof' yourself by always planning ahead, or 'blueprinting', and by familiarizing yourself with 'coping with setbacks' and 'changing your life-style' which come later in this section.

1. '*Blueprinting*'. This exercise is also known as 'trouble shooting'. It requires you to set some time aside for thinking about your future challenges and identifying where and when you will be vulnerable to stress. You might list: 'Giving a brief presentation to colleagues about my work' or 'Taking this faulty iron back to the shop' or 'Going into the garden shed, which has spiders inside'. Have a go at identifying your challenges for the next week.

Once you have predicted those situations which will be stressful, plan how you will deal with the challenge. Think how you might prepare yourself by relaxing and by rehearsing before you are in the situation and plan how you will deal with the stress when you face it. Which of your coping techniques will help you? Consider how you will deal with the situation if everything does not go according to plan—have a back-up scheme.

By now, you should be very familiar with your personal areas of difficulty and your own vulnerabilities. List the situations which you will probably find difficult in the future and then make a corresponding list of solutions.

Situations which I will find difficult **My coping strategy (ies).**

1. ....

2. ....

3. ....

4. ....

5. ....

2. *Coping with set-backs*. You will, from time to time, be disappointed in your performance and then it is important to:

- Accept that slips, or set-backs are to be expected. A *lapse* in your progress does not necessarily mean *collapse*.
- Recognize that a set-back is also a learning opportunity: what have you learnt about yourself that you can compensate for next time?
- Make a plan for tackling the problem again.

3. *Changing your life-style*. There are simple modifications which you can make in your day to day routines which will further 'stress proof' you in the future.

- Build a 'relaxation slot' into your daily routine. This might only be a few minutes but it will be a valuable use of your time. Try to develop the habit of relaxing.
- Do as many pleasurable things as possible. All the better if your pleasurable activities release tension, too. You might try physical exercise and yoga.
- Don't let stress build up. If something is worrying you, seek advice from friends or professionals. Find out now where you might seek help—have a list of useful telephone numbers, which will include friends and organizations such as the Samaritans.
- Organize yourself at home and at work. If you need professional help, find a time management course in your area.
- Assert yourself at home and at work. Avoid the unnecessary stress of being exploited. Look out for local assertiveness training classes or search the library for books on this topic.
- Avoid getting overtired or taking on too much. Recognize when you have reached your limit and stop. Take a break and try to do something relaxing and/or pleasurable.

- Don't avoid what you fear. If you find something is becoming difficult for you to face up to, don't back away because that situation will only grow more frightening. Instead, set yourself a series of small and safe steps to help you meet the challenge.
- Remember to recognize your achievements and to praise yourself. Never downgrade yourself and don't dwell on past difficulties. Plan and look ahead.

Dealing with problems

Dependency: It is possible that your client will continue to look to you for help rather than trying to be independent. Some professionals, such as the GP, are in a particularly difficult position when it comes to dependency because they are always available for consultation and thus the dependent client always has access.

The likelihood of dependency can be minimized if, from the outset, it is made clear that AMT is a relatively brief intervention which is aimed at developing self-help skills. Be explicit in your expectation that the client will take on the role of therapist. Throughout therapy, hand over responsibility and reinforce all autonomous actions with praise. Replace 'we' statements with 'you' statements, asking questions like: 'What do you think?', 'What do you see as the solution?', 'Given your understanding of your problem, how are you going to go about facing this challenge?'

Set-backs: These are inevitable and are likely to occur during the period of anxiety management training. Set-backs are to be welcomed as they provide the opportunity to teach relapse prevention. From the outset, prepare the client for lapses and hiccups and encourage your client to ask 'What I can learn from this' as soon as possible after the event. At first, a client might have difficulty in viewing an unsuccessful venture as a learning experience, particularly if her or his thinking style is dichotomous, but this is an essential part of relapse prevention and no set-back should be dismissed without analysis. For this reason, it is beneficial if the disappointment occurs during therapy, then, the client and therapist can work together on resolution of the new problem. Set-backs are very likely to occur in the follow-up period and the final therapy session can usefully be given over to discussing their management.

The end of therapy: case examples

A case of generalized anxiety: Mrs Green

> At their final session, Mrs Green and her GP identified those times or situations where she was likely to be vulnerable to anxiety, such as when she had taken on too much work at the church and had become over-tired. They then worked out coping strategies for each situation, so that Mrs Green had a blueprint for coping independently.

When Mrs Green visited her GP 3 months after she had achieved her goal, she reported that she no longer felt herself to have a problem. She described her experience of anxiety as 'normal levels of tension which I can tolerate as it no longer frightens me'. She was also confident that when she did get over-tense, she could manage her own anxiety using relaxation and/or distraction. Since their last meeting, she had made several more journeys to Birmingham, and had even been to Scotland to see her daughter and grandchild. She was now much more socially active and had not taken a tranquillizer since she had initially sought help. She was even cutting down on her cigarette consumption.

Mrs Green felt that the 3-month period of independent coping had been very valuable as it had allowed her to practise her skills with the reassurance that she had a specific appointment with her GP to discuss any problems. Rather than rush to the surgery each time she had a minor set-back, she saved her questions for the follow-up session 3 months later. In this way she had worked without the direct support of the GP for a long enough time to gain confidence in herself.

A case of specific phobia: Mrs Smith

Two months after the incident which had brought her problem to the attention of the health visitor, Mrs Smith invited her therapist to her eldest child's birthday party. This took place in the garden and featured much sugary food which attracted the odd wasp. Although Mrs Smith felt some apprehension when a wasp came into view, she was able to control her anxiety, and enjoy the party.

She was continuing to shop at the greengrocer's and leave the house windows open. She had also noticed that her aversion to being touched had almost disappeared. When asked what she had found most helpful, she said that the formulation had made a huge difference in how she saw her problem, and had given her hope that she could overcome it. She also stressed the importance of the encouragement she had received from the health visitor. She recognized that she tended to devalue her progress as she moved towards her goals, and the health visitor's reinforcement reminded her that she was making progress and boosted her confidence.

A case of panic attacks: Mr Peters

Mr Peters did try to move up the hierarchy too swiftly and had a very bad panic attack on the motorway on his way back from work. He then avoided driving until his next session with the nurse. Two important developments were made in this session. First, in analysing the event, Mr Peters was able to practise learning from set-backs. He discovered more about his personal vulnerabilities to stress and was able to view his panic attack, not as a 'failure', but as an indication that he had tried to tackle too difficult a task when he was feeling emotionally fragile. On the morning before this recent panic, he had had a row with his ex-wife. Secondly, his heightened tension following the row highlighted the fact that Mr Peters still held much unresolved anger for his first wife, and discussing this led to his also recognizing his unexpressed feelings about his father's death. For the first time, Mr Peters had acknowledged these emotions.

He went on to complete the hierarchy of tasks in only a few weeks, and agreed that it would be helpful if he were referred to the practice counsellor for help in coming to terms with his father's death and the failure of his first marriage.

Three months later, he met the practice nurse and proudly announced that he had not had another panic attack since the one on the motorway. He had gained his former confidence about driving and was much less concerned about his health. Over the 12 weeks that he had taken full responsibility for managing his own therapy, he had come to appreciate the importance of pacing his work-load so that he did not get over-tired and thus become vulnerable to excessive tension. He also revealed that he had grown less inhibited about expressing emotions, which meant that he now discussed his worries with colleagues or with his wife, rather than keeping them to himself. He felt that the combination of behaviour therapy, followed by counselling had been just what he needed.

A case of obsessional–compulsive behaviour: Mr Oldham

In their final treatment session, the CPN helped Mr Oldham to plan for future coping, by assisting him in drawing up a list of times and situations when Mr Oldham predicted he would find it difficult to resist checking. They then generated a list of solutions or coping strategies for such situations. The most important aspect of this was helping Mr Oldham accept that he would have set-backs and difficult times, but that they were part of normal progress, not an indication of failure.

The CPN contracted Mr Oldham once more, for a follow-up visit after 3 months. By this time the obsessional behaviour was no longer a problem. There had been one or two occasions when Mr Oldham had carried out an extra safety check, but he was prepared for this because he was aware of his times of vulnerability. As a consequence, he had not dwelt on the set-backs, but tried to learn from them. He said that he had been most helped by developing a better understanding of his problem, which had highlighted a need to talk about his worries more. He now discussed his troubles with his wife, who was invariably extremely helpful. By then discussing his concerns about not coping at work with his boss, he discovered that he had misunderstood his new duties and had actually taken on more responsibility than he should have. This was rectified and he began to enjoy his job once more.

A case of PTSD: Mr Thomas

Mr Thomas overcame his fearful images of his road traffic accident within a week or two of starting treatment and was confident about driving within 3 months. He and his counsellor then tried to identify when he was likely to be vulnerable to distress in the future. Both felt that his greatest vulnerability was his low self-esteem and Mr Thomas was offered sessions with the community-based clinical psychologist who was able to take him on for brief cognitive therapy which would focus on this. He also realized that, if he felt tired or stressed or hungry, he tended to persuade his wife to drive and that it then became more difficult for him to take the wheel again. Therefore, he resolved not to avoid and to make this easier for himself by not getting over-stressed.

Flashbacks no longer bothered him, but he was occasionally disturbed by a nightmare relating car accidents. He was now able to link these with times of stress and to accept that the process of recovery from PTSD might take longer than a month or two.

A case of executive stress: Dr Evans

At 3 month follow-up, Dr Evans was continuing to monitor and manage her stress. The Paris conference had gone well and she had only one set-back when her enthusiasm for excitement caused her to take on too much socially and this began to undermine her work. She found that she needed to keep some form of daily stress and performance log as a reminder of the benefits of pacing herself and so she designed one for her personal organizer which went with her everywhere.

From the case examples, it is evident that AMT is sometimes only part of a wider treatment programme and that it can be usefully supplemented by counselling, psychotherapy, or further skills training. Useful adjuncts to the basic AMT programme are guidelines for tranquillizer withdrawal and advice on improving sleep patterns. These appear in the appendices (Appendices 2 and 3, respectively) along with brief overviews of assertiveness (Appendix 4) and time management (Appendix 5). The latter benefit most of us, particularly those with anxiety-related problems, and clients can further help themselves by joining courses run by their organizations or community-based classes. Client Information Sheets 10 and 11 can be used to introduce the basic techniques and benefits of assertiveness and time management training.

15 *Summary of Part III: Working with your client*

Summary of Chapter 11: Anxiety

1. Present your client with the option of AMT. Obtain feedback and give written information about anxiety and AMT.
2. Present your client with the rationale for AMT. Emphasize that anxiety is normal and can be controlled but not cured. Present your formulation of the problem to the client. Make your management plan specific to your client's resources.
3. Establish a good working relationship, enlisting your client as a collaborator in therapy. Make your aims clear to your client, and get feedback.
4. Set homework and make a specific appointment.

Summary of Chapter 12: Control

1. Prepare your client by outlining the principles of self-management:
   - Control not cure;
   - anticipation and preparation;
   - repeated practice.
2. Choose your technique(s) from the following.
   - Relaxation: rationale
practical session if possible
diary if necessary
set homework
   - Controlled breathing: rationale
practical session if possible
diary if necessary
set homework

- Thought management: rationale
  diary
  rehearse
  set homework

- Panic management: rationale and reassurance
  controlled breathing if necessary
  emphasize practice in relaxation and thought management

3. Use information sheets as a supplement.

Summary of Chapter 13: Dealing with avoidance

1. Give the rationale for graded practice. Provide an information sheet.
2. Select specific, realistic targets and rank them. Choose one target.
3. Reduce the target into a hierarchy of small, specific, graded tasks. Take one task at a time.
4. Practise and record.
5. Build on success and prepare your client for set-backs.
6. Transfer responsibility for graded exposure to your client.

Summary of Chapter 14: Self-management and ending therapy

1. Review progress. Having decided to end therapy, give your client advance warning.
2. Prepare for termination by *blueprinting* and eliciting your client's worries about coping alone.
3. Discuss the management of set-backs.
4. Fix a follow-up appointment.

PART IV

Appendices

Appendix 1: *Group work*

It has been established that, with certain clients, fears can be treated successfully in a group setting (Robinson and Suinn 1969; Wolpe 1985; Telch *et al.* 1993). This approach saves time for the therapist and also has benefits for the participant, the most obvious of these being peer support, vicarious learning, and the destigmatizing of anxiety-related problems.

Anxiety management groups are probably best run as a course lasting for a finite number of sessions and following a set programme. This means that group members are all at the same stage in training and their shared experiences are meaningful to one another. Some useful guidelines for running groups are given below.

Preparation All potential participants should be assessed individually, prior to their admission to the group. It is useful to aim for a degree of homogeneity and to eliminate those who are likely to disrupt the cohesion of the group. Candidates who would be unsuitable for working with or in front of others might be those who express a fear or resistance to working in a group, or who have idiosyncratic or complex problems and so have little in common with other members. In these instances, other forms of therapy can be considered.

It is advisable to have a set programme for the course. A specimen outline of a six-session group is printed at the end of this section. Each of these sessions lasts about 90 minutes.

Numbers The number of members will depend on the number of therapists involved, and the size of the premises available. Between six and eight participants has been suggested as the optimum size if there is one main therapist (Wolpe 1985).

Co-therapists It can be very helpful to have more than one group leader, who can observe and evaluate the group and who can act as another discussant in this setting. A co-therapist can also be involved in leading subgroup tasks. The role of the co-therapist should always be established before the group starts.

The initial session(s) In the first session(s) the therapist(s) should present the programme for the course. Members can be invited to introduce themselves, but it might be worrying for some of the participants to have to reveal their problems to the rest of the group, so this could be left up to them.

An early sub-goal is the development of group cohesion, and the early sessions can be crucial for the development of a sense of shared commitment. You can try to enhance this by involving everyone in the group activities without putting pressure on anyone to perform. People need to feel safe and valued in the group if they are going to choose to stay.

Start by providing members with information about the psychological model of anxiety and its management. This can be in the form of teaching, supplemented by an information sheet. The early session(s) might usefully incorporate an introduction to relaxation training, followed by group relaxation practice. This can be done using a tape or spoken instruction. If time allows, subsequent sessions should include practical relaxation.

From the first meeting, members need to be set homework in the form of diary keeping and practising their coping skills regularly. People are more likely to cooperate with homework assignments if set specific tasks. Keeping a diary and practising relaxation needs to be set as homework at the end of every session, at least in the early stages of the group.

Below is an example of an AMT group programme and an indication of the possible content of the first two sessions.

An introduction to the self-management of anxiety: Group work

Therapist: 'The purpose of this group is to help you to learn ways of coping with your feelings of anxiety, tension, and stress. There will be six sessions, designed to get you started on your way towards controlling your own anxieties. The real ''work'' is done by you, outside the sessions. You will need to practise regularly and carry out homework tasks in order to feel the benefit of these meetings. The programme is as follows:

Week 1: introduction;
Week 2: how to relax;

Week 3: breathing properly;
Week 4: facing fears;
Week 5: coping with worrying thoughts;
Week 6: coping in the long term.'

Example of week 1: introduction to AMT

1. Introduction

Begin with a structured introduction of group members. Give clear guidelines on what each is expected to disclose. Keep anxiety low! Introduce the function of the group. Run through the programme, including homework tasks, and invite questions.

2. Assessment

Administer an anxiety checklist at an early stage (e.g. Beck *et al.* 1986).

3. Teaching

Introduce the idea of 'normal anxiety'. Elicit symptoms of anxiety from the group and structure them as follows: *somatic* symptoms; *behavioural* symptoms; *cognitive* symptoms. Discuss how these affect members and how anxiety might be mistaken for a physical illness, such as having a heart attack. Also, discuss ways of dealing with symptoms, identifying the *adaptive* and *maladaptive* strategies. Finally, introduce the concept of AMT and the skills which will be learnt in the group. Invite questions and give out Client Information Sheet 1.

4. Homework

This could be to read the information handout and keep a record of anxiety levels using Diary 1. Explain the rationale and method of diary keeping and check that all members understand.

Example of week 2: relaxation training

1. Assessment

Administer the anxiety check-list.

2. Review

Review the diaries, focusing on *patterns* of behaviours and coping skills. Make sure that members are keeping diaries properly.

3. Teaching or practical

Members could work in pairs, discussing their physical symptoms. The therapist might then introduce the principle of physical relaxation followed by a practice relaxation exercise. Feedback should be invited and a training tape offered, if possible. Give out Client Information Sheet 2.

4. Homework

This could be to continue keeping an anxiety diary and to practise relaxation once or twice a day.

Subsequent sessions

Begin subsequent sessions with a review of the diaries and a group discussion focusing on the problem(s) and coping technique(s) which have been experienced by the group members. The depth of inquiry devoted to each person will depend on the size of the group and time available. It is very important to elicit any problems that members might be experiencing with stress control techniques, so that they can be dealt with before they present any real handicap for that person.

It is useful to organize your course such that each session focuses on a particular topic, with homework assignments relating to this. The minimum requirements are probably:

1. The role of muscular tension in anxiety. Homework assignment—relaxation practice.

2. The role of breathing in the development and maintenance of anxiety. Homework assignment—breathing exercises.

3. The role of irrational thoughts and beliefs in causing and maintaining fear. Homework assignment—distraction, rational thinking.

4. The function of graded practice and problem solving. Homework assignment—graded exposure in real-life situations.

Clearly, some topics may require more than one session. This again will depend on the size, needs, and receptiveness of the group, as well as the time available. The information given in sessions should be supplemented by the relevant information sheets.

Final session

The last meeting of any group should include:

1. A review and discussion of the homework and progress.

2. A review of the anxiety management strategies which have been covered in the course. It might be useful to summarize these in a written handout for group members.

3. Blueprinting, which means helping members to identify potential problem times or situations, and to generate coping strategies.

4. Gathering feedback from the group, both positive and negative. This information can be used constructively when setting up the next group.

Possible additions to the basic programme

If time permits, other topics, relating to anxiety control, can be incorporated into the group programme. For example, one or two sessions might be given over to assertiveness training, the principles of meditation, or the role of physical exercise. The best rule is to try to meet the needs of your group members as far as possible.

Appendix 2: *Medication*

Prescribing tranquillizers

Over the past few years, increasing concern has been expressed about the use of tranquillizers in the management of anxiety-related problems (See Catalan and Gath 1985 for a review) and there is evidence that medication regimens with benzodiazepines have resulted in weak and short-lived clinical improvement (Schweizer and Rickels 1991). Concern among medical practitioners has been paralleled by an increase in public awareness and a growing demand for tranquillizer reduction (Lacey and Woodward 1985). Support groups for tranquillizer withdrawal ('Tranx' groups) are being set up nation-wide, and it is likely that GPs will be faced with more and more patients wishing to come off their tranquillizers. Anxiety management training is useful in helping people reduce their use of tranquillizers.

The use of tranquillizers is not necessarily a bad thing and a doctor should prescribe anxiolytic medication as is appropriate. Tranquillizers can be helpful as a temporary means of coping with an acute problem. They can also be useful diagnostically, in that a positive response to tranquillizers could indicate that a problem is indeed one of anxiety and not organic.

However, problems can arise if treatment begins with the prescription of anxiolytics, as the client may then believe that the drugs will 'cure' the problem, and that anxiety management will be a passive procedure for them. It should be stressed that drugs are only a temporary means of support, as dependence can develop after only a few weeks. The client should be reassured that short-term use of anxiolytic medication is not harmful but that long-term use might result in dependency, and that while drugs are being relied upon for relief, the user is not developing innate coping mechanisms.

When necessary, give arguments against prescribing drugs. For example, medication masks symptoms but does not deal with the original causes of the problem; drugs have side-effects such as drowsiness, appetite changes, constipation, dry mouth, dizziness, and dependency, and therefore can actually exacerbate one's problems; the problems which will eventually have to be faced are the consequence of real life, not a medical condition, so drugs are not the answer; personal coping resources can be sufficient to deal with problems if the client is trained in self-help skills.

If tranquillizers are prescribed, Tyrer and Murphy (1987) suggest some useful guidelines. They advise that benzodiazepines should not be prescribed for more than a 2-week period, that drugs with a short half-life should be avoided and, when a patient is given a medication for more than a fortnight, this should be on an intermittent or flexible basis.

Withdrawal from tranquillizers

When working with a client with a view to ceasing medication, it is important to be aware of the possible withdrawal effects. Withdrawal symptoms are not necessarily a consequence of long-term use of medication, but have been reported after only a few weeks of use (Higgitt *et al.* 1985). The symptoms typically emerge in the first week after stopping the drug, but may become apparent after a reduction in dosage. If a person is reducing benzodiazepine use, some 'anxiety' symptoms may be withdrawal symptoms, and increasing the dose would be counter-productive. Common withdrawal symptoms are:

anxiety
loss of confidence
agitation
pins and needles
palpitations
restlessness
loss of appetite
gastrointestinal upset
trembling
hypersensitivity to light, touch, and noise
feelings of unreality
muscular tension
panic attacks
sweating
shaking
headache
aches and pains
nausea
insomnia
lack of concentration and poor memory.

Therapy can be aimed at reducing symptoms relating to the original anxiety, as well as reducing those which are a consequence of withdrawal. Special care should also be taken to identify complications of withdrawal, such as increased alcohol consumption and smoking, or the development of interpersonal and social problems.

The optimum reduction rate varies with different drugs. In general, the faster the substance is metabolized, the more gradual should be its reduction and the longer the use of tranquillizers, the slower the withdrawal rate (Tyrer 1984).

Lader (1984) suggests the following minimum-time withdrawal plan, but practitioners might well consider slower rates of reduction.

≤ 15 mg Valium/day (or equivalent): reduce over 5 weeks;
15–30 mg Valium/day (or equivalent): reduce over 6 weeks;
≥ 30 mg Valium/day (or equivalent): reduce over 6 + weeks.

Lader stresses that this is the shortest time which should be allowed for withdrawal, and recommends that the reduction be by equal parts each week. It is important to note what is happening in your client's life during the withdrawal period, as extra stress or tensions at this time might require a temporary cessation in drug reduction.

During the period of tranquillizer reduction, your client may experience 'psychological withdrawal', that is, distress and heightened anxiety because of a loss of confidence in the ability to cope without medication. In these instances successful withdrawal might take longer than Lader suggests, as the person will need time to build up a sense of self-confidence.

It is common for a practitioner to change short-acting benzodiazepines to an equivalent dose of the longer half-life variety or to change to beta-blockers before instructing someone to cut down on medication. Alternatively, a tricyclic or 5HT blocking antidepressant might be chosen by the GP or psychiatrist to ease the discomfort of tranquillizer withdrawal. Some GPs prescribe tranquillizers in liquid form so that the very small doses required in the latter stages of withdrawal can be more easily taken.

The client should be advised about the management of the withdrawal symptoms, as this is likely to render the symptoms less alarming. You can use Client Information Sheet 8 on page 000 to help your client remember the important details concerning tranquillizer use and withdrawal.

Most difficulties relating to withdrawal can be dealt with through reassurance and practical advice, whether this comes from a health professional or from participation in a 'Tranx' group. During the period of drug reduction, people often attribute almost all physical and psychological changes to withdrawal effects. If inappropriate, this view should be corrected and the client helped to understand the real source of the symptoms of anxiety.

Client information sheet 8: **Coming off tranquillizers**

Learning to control your feelings of anxiety, by yourself, can be an alternative to tranquilizers. Self-management of anxiety can also be used to help you to reduce tranquillizer use.

There are good reasons for avoiding or decreasing your use of tranquillizers.

1. Tranquillizers often have physical side-effects, such as dizziness, headache, drowsiness, and poor co-ordination. These can be as disturbing as the feelings of anxiety which you are trying to avoid.

2. Using tranquillizers sometimes makes it easier to avoid dealing with the real problem. If they are regarded as a 'medicine' for an illness, it becomes difficult to accept that control of anxiety can lie with you. In addition, tranquillizers dull the emotions, making it easier to put off tackling problems which exist or may arise.

3. Bodily or mental dependence can develop in some people. This makes coming off tranquillizers very unpleasant.

The *bodily* effects of withdrawal include:

palpitations
sleeplessness
aches and pains
restlessness
headache
over-sensitivity to noise, touch, and light.
pins and needles
loss of appetite
trembling
sweating
feelings of sickness

The *mental* effects are:

feelings of anxiety
loss of confidence
poor concentration and memory.
tension
feelings of unreality

Not everyone has these feelings when they stop using tranquillizers, but it is important to be aware of the temporary changes which you might experience. It is also important to recognize that these feelings *are not* the original anxiety returning, although some of the symptoms may be similar. Difficulty in sleeping is a common complaint during tranquillizer withdrawal. Don't worry about this, it is part of your progress and will improve if you relax about it.

You can successfully withdraw from tranquillizers with the help of your GP who will decrease your dose at a safe speed. Alternatively, you can come off tranquillizers by joining a 'Tranquillizer Withdrawal Support Group'. You can get the details of your local group from: MIND, The National Association for Mental Health, Granta House 15–19 Broadway Stratford London E15 4BQ.

Coming off tranquillizers is not always easy; it is usual to have difficult times when it is very hard to cope. When this happens, remember:

Take one day at a time Think that you are coping with—'just today', because looking ahead to a life without tranquillizers can be too alarming. If things get very difficult, think of facing one hour at a time or even a minute at a time until your crisis has passed.

Talk to yourself Give yourself encouragement. Think of what you would say to a friend under stress and then say this to yourself. Tell yourself about the disadvantages of taking tranquillizers and plan for your life without them.

Talk to others There is no need to be ashamed of tranquillizer withdrawal. You might find that sharing your experience with others helps you to cope.

Keep busy Keeping active and occupied can take your mind off stress.

Keep a diary Note all positive effects of not taking tranquillizers and of each 'good day' since you began to withdraw. Looking back over this can help you feel more optimistic during a difficult time.

Use your anxiety management skills Remember to put into practice relaxing and controlling your worrying thoughts when you are very stressed. The more you use these techniques, the better you will become at controlling your own anxiety and the less you will need tranquillizers.

Eventually you will regain confidence in your own ability to cope with stress.

Appendix 3: *Coping with insomnia*

Sleep disturbance is frequently associated with anxiety, and it has been estimated that 20 per cent of those who attend general practice complain of some degree of insomnia (Shepherd *et al.* 1981). Typically, a person will experience difficulty in getting off to sleep, broken sleep, or early morning wakening, the latter often being associated with depression rather than anxiety. The complainer's worry about the sleep pattern frequently exacerbates the problem.

Your client might well expect to take 8 hours sleep a night, not realizing that many people function efficiently on much less, and not appreciating that they are likely to require less sleep as they get older. Your client might also expect an unbroken period of sleep, while it is quite usual to drift into and out of sleep throughout the night. Most of us simply do not register this waking, but if these times are attended to and cause concern, it is very likely that the wakefulness will persist.

In short, worrying about the sleep patterns frequently underlies sleep problems. The first step which the professional can take in helping the client is to provide information about normal sleep patterns. Client Information Sheet 9 on page 000 contains useful details for someone who is worried about sleep patterns.

The next step is to establish whether your client's sleep pattern is abnormal, and whether this impairs performance in any way. Although we know that sleep deprivation can result in acute emotional changes and impairment of memory and task performance (Carlson 1977), this is usually the result of extreme sleep loss whereas most clients will only complain of minor sleep loss. The best way of finding out how much sleep your client is getting and how this affects performance, is to suggest that a sleep diary is kept. This should contain the following information:

- date and any significant events of that day;
- hours of sleep and number of waking episodes recalled;
- coping strategies and their effectiveness;

Client information sheet 9: **Coping with sleep problems**

Sleep problems are common. As many as one in five people complains of difficulty in falling asleep, of waking too frequently throughout the night, or of early morning wakening. These experiences are quite normal and only become a problem when you worry about them. Worry, more than anything else, will keep you awake.

The worries can be more unpleasant and undermining than the lack of sleep itself and can exhaust you just as much. To help you to minimize worrying, here are some facts about sleep which are useful to know are:

1. There is no such thing as the ideal length of sleep: some people need 10 hours and some need 3. If you sleep less than 8 hours a night, you are not necessarily depriving your body of sleep—you might not need 8 hours. It is said that Napoleon and Churchill only slept for 3 or 4 hours a night.
2. As you grow older, you will require less sleep.
3. Everyone has 'broken sleep' in that we all wake several times during the night, and simply go back to sleep. It is only when you worry about this happening that you stay awake.
4. There is no danger in losing a few nights of 'good sleep'. Everyone experiences periods of poor sleeping, especially when under stress. The only effect of this is that you will feel more sleepy and/or irritable during the day until you re-establish a good sleeping pattern.
5. Sleep is affected by many things; stress, mood, exercise, food, medicines, alcohol. By altering your behaviour you can take control of your sleeping pattern without resorting to drugs.

Why avoid drugs?

Sleeping tablets are addictive. An occasional sleeping pill, taken on your doctor's advice, might be useful in the short-term. However, your body quickly comes to rely on them and very soon it is difficult to sleep without medication. When you try to stop taking them, you can find that your sleep pattern is worse than ever and that you want to revert to taking the pills. This can start a cycle of poor sleep and turning to drugs.

Coping without drugs

Fortunately, you can learn to overcome sleep problems without taking tablets, simply by altering your behaviour. The first thing to do is to find out more about your sleep pattern, which means keeping a sleep diary. All you need to do is to record the following details for a week or two:

1. The date and any events which may affect your sleep: e.g. what food you ate before going to bed, how much stress you were under, what exercise you took, etc.
2. How many hours of sleep you had and how many waking episodes you recalled.
3. What you did when you could not sleep, e.g. made a cup of tea, read, etc. Make a note as to whether this helped or not.
4. How alert or awake you felt the next day. You can rate yourself on a 10-point scale, where 1 is extremely dull and 10 is very alert.
5. How well you think you carried out your work the next day. Again, you can rate yourself on a 10-point scale, where 1 is very badly and 10 is very well.

When you have kept a diary, you can see whether or not you have a problem. If you are feeling reasonably alert and working reasonably well on your usual number of hours' sleep, then you don't have a problem. If you are feeling tired and your work is suffering, then you can start to help yourself by trying the following:

1. Relax: remember, no one has unbroken sleep and everyone has the odd period of poor sleep. If you don't worry, you will sleep better.
2. Prepare yourself before going to bed. This will involve:
   (a) taking exercise earlier in the day;
   (b) avoiding spicy or heavy food and caffeine in the few hours before you retire;
   (c) having a milky drink (not cocoa) before bed;

(d) taking time to relax by having a warm bath, listening to restful music, or completing a relaxation exercise.
(e) making sure your bedroom is quiet—secure rattling windows and doors;
(f) emptying your bladder;
(g) avoiding alcohol and nicotine in the hours before bedtime as they can act as a stimulant keeping you awake.

3. Go to bed only when you are sleepy, and only use your bed for sleeping. This means not eating or reading or watching television, etc. in bed.

4. When you are in bed, relax and do not think about worrying issues. Use your relaxation and distraction exercises to help you.

5. If you have not fallen asleep in about 15 minutes, or if you wake and have not fallen asleep again in 10–15 minutes, then get out of bed and do something else until you feel sleepy. Don't lie there tossing and turning.

6. Set an alarm so that you wake at a regular time each day. Get up when your alarm goes off and do not be tempted to cat-nap during the day or to sleep overlong at the weekend. For now, you are trying to establish good sleeping routine.

7. Look at your sleep diary. What helped you to get back to sleep? Try these techniques again and avoid the activities which did not help.

If you follow these suggestions and try to relax you will find that you have little difficulty in sleeping.

- alertness the following day (rate 1–10);
- competence in activities (rate 1–10).

Using this information, you can determine whether a particular sleep pattern is simply a normal response to life stress and thus likely to remit, or if it is within the normal range of sleeping patterns in which case intervention need only be reassurance. A formal sleep programme can be introduced when the sleep pattern is disturbed enough to impair cognitive functioning and/or affect. Diary 4, on page 202 is a typical sleep diary which you might find useful.

From the diary, you will also get an idea of what adaptive coping strategies work for your client. For example, an evening's physical exercise or a hot milky drink might help. You can then encourage these, while discouraging the maladaptive coping methods such as drinking alcohol before bed. Although one or two units of alcohol can promote sleep, it is metabolized quickly and results in a rebound period of increased arousal. Similarly, nicotine in small doses is sedative but becomes arousing as the amount increases (Stradling *et al.* 1993).

Why avoid sleeping pills?

According to Dement (1972), 'sleeping pills cause insomnia'. Most hypnotics lose their sleep-promoting property within 3–14 days of continuous use (Committee on the Review of Medicines 1980). Insomnia has been found to recur after only a few weeks of using benzodiazepine hypnotics (Kales *et al.* 1983). Carlson (1977) argues that sleeping medications do not induce normal sleep, and promote dependence. Initially they suppress D-sleep, which is characterized by dreaming, and allow the person to enter S-sleep which is a deeper sleep. This effect quickly habituates, an abnormal, dulled D-sleep re-emerges, and the medication seems less effective. The result of cessation of medication is a major recurrence of D-sleep, which is associated with vivid nightmares and sleeplessness. When this happens, the patient requires more pills in order to get to sleep again and dependency results. Fortunately, there is a psychological alternative to drug treatment.

The psychological alternative

Good sleeping habits can be re-established by attending to the following behavioural recommendations:

1. Going to bed only when sleepy and reserving bed for sleeping and not for watching TV, eating, or reading.
2. Using relaxation and distraction exercises on retiring and on premature wakening.
3. Getting up and doing something in another area if sleeplessness exceeds 10–15 minutes. Only returning to bed when sleepy, and repeating the exercise if necessary.
4. Setting the alarm for the same time each morning and always rising then. No cat-naps and no 'sleeping binges'.
5. Avoiding stimulants, especially caffeine, alcohol, nicotine, and spicy foods, at night.

The guidelines are elaborated upon in Client Information Sheet 9 (p. 176).

Other sleep problems

Your client may complain of other sleep worries which are distressing to him or her, but not harmful. Oswald (1962) reviews these in some detail, describing them as exaggerated normal phenomena. For example, a person may experience some of the following.

Sleep paralysis A temporary episode of wakefulness when one is unable to move. Usually this lasts for only a few seconds but it can be quite frightening. The reason for this experience is that the body is paralysed during D-sleep, while the brain remains active. During light sleep and drowsing the sleeper can become aware of this muscular flaccidity.

Sensory shocks These are most usually bodily sensations in the form of jerks, or the sensation of falling. Sensory shocks can also include auditory, visual, and olfactory sensation, which are sometimes vivid enough to wake the sleeper.

Hypnogogic and hypnopompic hallucinations There occur as a person falls asleep or wakes, respectively. It is the state of half-sleep when fleeting but vivid images are common, and sometimes frightening.

Again, you can reassure your client that none of these experiences is harmful and that relaxing and accepting them is the best coping strategy.

Parasomnias such as *sleepwalking*, which can be dangerous to the sufferer, and *night terrors* can often be helped by psychotherapy or hypnosis (Driver and Shapiro 1993) and therefore a referral to a specialist might best help the client.

Appendix 4: *How to assert yourself*

Assertiveness is an interpersonal skill. It describes a way of communicating your *needs*, your *wants* and your *feelings* to others without infringing their rights. It means acknowledging your own rights whilst respecting the rights of others.

Personal rights

Before you can assert yourself, you need to be aware of your personal rights such as the right to:

Say: 'No' without feeling guilty.

Change your mind.

Make mistakes and be responsible for them.

Say: 'I don't know', 'I don't understand', 'I don't care'.

Ask a person for what you want, while realizing that person has the right to say 'No'.

Have opinions and feelings and the right to express them appropriately.

Choose whether or not to get involved in the problems of someone else.

The right to privacy.

Consider the rights which you intend to assert in the future.

Assertiveness

Being assertive means communicating in a way which is not passive, nor aggressive, nor manipulative. The goal of assertive behaviour is to confront without undermining oneself or others, while the goal of passivity is to avoid conflict, and the goal of aggressive or manipulative behaviour is to win. Passivity and aggression are easy to spot, but the manipulative person is less easy to recognize as an aggressor.

The *passive* type opts out of conflict, cannot make decisions and aims to please all of the people all of the time. This person respects the rights of others without regard for her or his own rights.

The *aggressive* type comes across loudly and forcefully, belittling the thoughts, actions, and personal qualities of others. He or she must win and disrespects others.

The *manipulative* type is indirectly aggressive and controlling but attack is concealed. This person may appear to be supportive and understanding, but uses emotional blackmail and subtly undermines the rights of others.

The *assertive* type accepts personal faults and strengths, respects personal needs, takes responsibility for his or her own actions—in the context of respecting others' rights. To be assertive you must:

decide what you *want*;

decide if it is *fair*;

ask for it *clearly*;

be prepared to take *risks*;

keep *calm*.

It is all very well knowing what 'being assertive' is, but you cannot put theory into practice if you are too stressed. So, use your anxiety management skills to help you to stay calm.

General guidelines

1. *Prepare yourself.* Brief yourself so that you know your arguments are sound. Your argument does not have to be elaborate to be sound—often, simple explanations and requests are most effective. Script your argument in advance and organize it in terms of: the *explanation*, your *feelings*, your *needs*, and the *consequences*.

For example:

The explanation: 'I want to discuss a problem with you. In the last few weeks, your conversations, in the office, with Mary seem to have increased. This has disturbed my concentration on several occasions and I find it difficult to do my work'.

Your feelings: 'Although I realize that we all need social contact and periodic breaks from work, I am now feeling irritated by it'.

Your needs: 'However, if you could talk more quietly or use the coffee room for conversation I would be able to get on with my work'.

The consequences: 'If not, I know my work will suffer'.

It can be useful to draft a script for yourself, then you can rehearse your arguments in advance. Try them out on a friend if necessary. The more confident you are, the more effective you will be in confrontation.

2. *Be positive*. A safe way of beginning is by using a compliment or a positive statement. For example, 'This is an excellent piece of work, but I would like you to write more clearly so that it is easier for me to read next time'. 'That is a very good idea, but I don't think that it would work here'.

3. *Be objective*. Do not get involved in personal criticism, but do explain the *situation* as you see it. Never criticize the person, only the behaviour.

4. *Be brief*. Avoid the other person switching off, butting in or side-tracking, by being succinct. Don't theorize, just describe the facts.

5. *Be aware of manipulative criticism*. Don't expect that the person with whom you are trying to assert yourself to be cooperative and concede to your point. He or she could try to undermine your efforts by using criticism such as: nagging, lecturing or insulting you or accusing you of upsetting them.

Specific techniques

There are three basic techniques:

1. *The broken record*. Unassertive people take 'no' for an answer far too easily. A basic assertiveness skill is being persistent and repeating what you want over and over again—calmly. You have decided that what you want to say is fair, so go ahead and assert it. Once you have prepared your 'script' you can relax and repeat your message until the other person accepts or agrees to negotiate with you. You know exactly what you are going to say, however abusive or manipulative the other person tries to be, and this will make it easier for you not to accept 'no'.

This is particularly useful when:

- Dealing with situations where your rights are clearly in danger of being abused.
- Coping with situations where you are likely to be diverted by articulate but irrelevant arguments.
- Situations where you feel vulnerable because you know the other person will use criticism to undermine your self-esteem.

2. *Fogging/fielding*. This will help you to deal with manipulative criticism—the sort that leaves you feeling bad about yourself so that you agree to do something which you would rather not. There is often an element of truth in what is being said, but this is exaggerated. For example: 'Typical! You're always late… insensitive… selfish… expect others to do your work…' might well trigger some guilt and a subsequent unassertive response. In fact, the only truth in the statement might be 'You are late'.

Fogging or fielding means calmly acknowledging that there may be some truth in what has been said: 'Yes, I am late'. It can be left at that, if you do not want to get more involved, or followed by a reassertion of your view. Fogging stops the manipulative criticism escalating into a personal argument and keeping the situation calm and buys you some time to think clearly.

3. *Negotiating*. The aim of being assertive is not to win at all costs, but to reach a solution which is reasonable to all parties. This will involve compromise and negotiation. Negotiating can be made easier by following these rules:

- Ask for *clarification* of the argument so that you understand the issue and are aware of the other person's position, reasoning, and needs.
- *Keep calm* by using controlled breathing and adopting a relaxed attitude.
- *Be prepared*: if you have time, do your homework—get the facts to support your case and rehearse your script.
- *Acknowledge the other side of the argument* ('I understand your position, but…'). Try to empathize.
- *Never attack* the whole person, only the behaviour with which you disagree.

- *Keep to the point*: don't get led away from your argument. Make your point and repeat yourself as often as is necessary.
- *Be prepared to compromise.* Do not be stubborn and determined to win—this is aggression! Decide in advance, how far you are prepared to compromise.

Being assertive isn't very difficult when you are aware of, and have practised, the strategies which we have covered. However, it is crucial to plan and rehearse while you are a novice, otherwise you will slip too easily into the position of aggressor, manipulator, or avoider.

Assertiveness is a skill and is usefully learnt as part of an experiential course. Find out if there are classes in your community or if your workplace organizes assertiveness training courses. You might also find the following books useful in broadening your understanding of assertiveness:

Dickson, A. (1982). *A woman in your own right*, Quartet Books.

Lindenfield, G. (1986). *Assert yourself*, Thorsons Publishing Group.

Smith, M. (1975). *When I say no, I feel guilty*, Bantam Books.

Appendix 5: *How to manage your time*

For many, learning to manage time efficiently reduces stress. This requires good organization and preparation and most people who fail at time management do so because they have neglected the groundwork prior to taking on a task, not because they have misunderstood the principles of time management. The groundwork involves appreciating ones priorities, ones resources, responsibilities and goals, and then planning task(s) around these.

1. *Priorities*. The first step, in time management, is taking stock of your values by listing all the important areas of your life: career; health; family; money, etc. Write down what means most to you and how much of your time you want to give to each of these areas.

Next, prioritize by ranking them according to importance or urgency (which ever is most appropriate at the time). Examples of priorities might be: getting the children to and from school on time; finishing an important project by a certain time; learning French. Then consider your task(s) in the context of your other priorities and be prepared to allocate only an appropriate amount of time to the task.

2. *Personal resources*. In order to manage *your* time efficiently, you need to be able to appraise yourself realistically and define your personal ***strengths*** and ***needs*** and design your time management plans around this. The sorts of questions to ask yourself are:

Do I plan ahead?
Do I prioritize?
Am I able to focus my concentration?
Am I punctual?
Do I put things off?
Do I make lists?
Do I work in a cluttered environment?
Can I say 'No'?
Do I conform/innovate?
Am I able to delegate?
Am I obsessional? a loner? a pessimist? empathic? a worrier?.......

Reflecting on these questions, you might conclude that your strengths are: you are a tidy and physically well organized person, but that you need to have diaries and wall charts around to keep you mentally organized; that you are flexible and can see others' points of view, but that you need to be careful not to conform too readily, and so on.

3. *Responsibilities.* It is crucial to be clear about your role(s) at home and at work. If this is fuzzy, you run the risk of taking on too much and/or letting down others. Ask yourself questions like: What are the main priorities of this family or this organization? What is it reasonable for me to I contribute? What are my basic responsibilities? What, therefore, are my realistic work tasks?

4. *Goals.* The next step is to refer to your task and set goals for achieving it without undermining other important areas of your life. For example, in doing charity work, do not neglect the family; in helping others in your organization, don't lose sight of your own needs for career development. Learn to compromise and to rethink your goals regularly.

When defining your goal, remember that a goal needs to be realistic and specific: who, what, when, how much, etc., must be spelt out clearly. For example, the goal: 'To be a better time keeper' is too vague. A better definition would be: *To arrive at work no later than 8.45 a.m. on busy days and no later than 9.00 a.m. during less busy periods; to take a lunch break between 12.30 and 1.00 p.m., which should last at least 30 minutes; to leave the office by 5.30 p.m. when business is quiet, but never later than 6.30 p.m. when we are busy.* This goal is unambiguous, so it is difficult to bend the rules without having to acknowledge that one is doing so. It is also easy to appreciate when the goal has been achieved. The goal recognizes personal needs for breaks during the day and, perhaps, time spent with the family.

Sometimes, goals can be achieved in one step: the revision of a diary can achieve certain time management goals at once or a single telephone call can attain a goal. However, some goals need more planning. Try to recognize when the attainment of a goal requires more than one step—if you don't and you expect to reach your target by a single action, you are setting yourself up for failure. If a target seems overwhelming, you are very likely to procrastinate unless you reduce the goal to several manageable steps. This might sound very laborious, but remember that good preparation and planning save time (and stress) in the long run; and with repeated application, this approach will become second nature.

Now you are in a position to schedule time in your diary for necessary tasks and to establish priorities. This analysis of tasks is best carried out each day and, with practice, can become part of your daily routine.

Organizing your time

Keeping a time record

Before you can start to mange your time better, you need to know what you do with it now by keeping a detailed diary for a sample period of time, every 15 minutes in a typical week, for example. In this way, you can see when you are most and least productive. Once you know how you spend your time, you can begin to reorganize your schedule for greater efficiency. In analysing your diary ask:

What do I do that is necessary to achieve my goals? Then give yourself credit.
What do I do that wastes time? Then plan to minimize these activities.
What do I do that others could handle instead? Then plan to delegate.

Daily organization

When you have identified the necessary tasks in your day, subdivide them again according to *importance*, which will determine how much time you give that task, and *urgency*, which should dictate how soon it is carried out. Allocate time, each day, to do this.

Delegation

You can give others responsibility for certain tasks, for example, you could delegate your spouse to do the weekly shopping; delegate an office task to your secretary; get your children to take in the washing and so on. Delegating might mean your giving up some things which you like doing, but it is necessary for effective time management.

Delegating requires you to be clear about the task to be delegated and to allocate to a suitable and capable person. It is often necessary to invest some time briefing and guiding the relevant person. Try not to give into thoughts such as: 'It's easier to do it myself', 'It's faster to do it myself', 'If you want a good job doing, do it yourself', 'I haven't the time to show her how to do it', 'At the end of the day, I'm responsible', because good delegation does save time and stress.

Delegation will fail if the delegee is not supported and monitored, but you do need to hand over the responsibility and authority for doing the job, otherwise you remain so involved that you are not economizing on time. It is also important to remember that delegation is not an excuse for passing on all the boring or unrewarding tasks.

This appendix can only give an impression of what is involved in time management. If you think that learning time management skills will help you better manage your anxiety, find out if your company runs courses or if there are evening classes available in your community. You could also try reading some of the many self-help texts on the market. Below are a few which you might find useful:

Bird, M. (1982). *The time effective manager*, Ebury Press.

Taylor, H. L. (1981). *Making time work for you: a guide book to effective and productive time management*, General.

Turla, P and Hawkins, K. L. (1985). *Time management made easy*, Panther Granada.

Appendix 6: *Instructions for making relaxation tapes*

Introduction

Relaxation training is often easier with guided instruction in the form of taped directions. Below are scripts which can be used by the therapist to make personal audio tapes.

Opening guidelines

'When any of us is anxious or stressed, the muscles in our body grow tense. The most effective way of controlling this bodily tension is by relaxing the muscles. However, the ability to relax is not always something which comes naturally, it is a skill which needs to be learnt. The following exercises are designed to help you learn how to relax. The first exercise is quite lengthy, but once it is effective for you, you can begin to shorten your relaxation routine until you reach the point when you can relax quite quickly. This will take time and cannot be rushed.'

General guidelines

'In advance, decide where you are going to practise. Make sure that you choose somewhere quiet, and that no one will disturb you. Don't try the exercise if you are hungry or have just eaten, as this will make it more difficult for you to relax. Similarly, don't use a room which is too hot or too chilly. It is important than you start by being as comfortable as possible. At first it might be helpful to do the exercises lying down in a comfortable position; later, you can practise while sitting or while walking around. It is very important to adopt what might be called "a passive attitude". That is, don't worry about your performance or whether you are relaxing properly. Don't be determined to relax, just have a go and see what happens. Try to breathe through your nose and use your stomach muscles as you inhale and exhale. Breathe slowly and regularly. It is important not to take a lot of quick deep breaths, as this can make you feel dizzy or faint, and even worsen your tension. It is useful to practise this rhythmic breathing before you begin the relaxation exercise, just to get used to the sensation. Try it now…'

Exercise 1: Progressive muscular relaxation or deep relaxation

'This exercise will help you to distinguish between tension and relaxation in your muscles, and teach you how to relax at will. We will work through various muscle groups, first tensing them and then relaxing them. We will start with your feet, then work up through your body slowly and smoothly. Try not to rush, just let the sensation of relaxation deepen at its own pace.

'First, make yourself as comfortable as you can … Lie flat on the floor with a pillow under your head, or snuggle in your chair … If you wear spectacles, remove them … Kick off your shoes and loosen any tight clothing … Relax your arms by your side and have your legs uncrossed … Close your eyes, and don't worry if they flicker—this is quite usual.

'You are now beginning to relax … Breathe out slowly … Now, breathe in smoothly and deeply … Now, breathe out slowly again, imagining yourself becoming heavier and heavier, sinking into the floor or your chair … Keep breathing rhythmically, and feel a sense of relief and of letting go … Try saying "relax" to yourself as you breathe out … Breathe like this for a few moments more….

'Now, we are going to begin to tense and relax the muscles of your body … Think of your feet … Tense the muscles in your feet and ankles, curling your toes towards your head … Gently stretch your muscles … Feel the tension in your feet and ankles … Hold it … Now let go … Let your feet go limp and floppy … Feel the difference … Feel the tension draining away from your feet … Let your feet roll outwards and grow heavier and heavier … Imagine that they are so heavy that they are sinking into the floor … More and more relaxed … growing heavier and more relaxed….

(Repeat)

'Now, think about your calves … Begin to tense the muscles in your lower legs … If you are sitting, lift your legs up and hold them in front of you, feeling the tension ... Gently stretch the muscles ... Feel the tension ... Hold it ... Now release ... Let your feet touch the floor and let your legs go floppy and heavy ... Feel the difference ... Feel the tension leaving your legs, draining from your calves ... Leaving your calves feeling heavy ... Draining away from your feet ... Leaving them feeling heavy and limp ... Imagine that your legs and feet are so heavy that they are sinking into the floor ... They feel limp and relaxed ... Growing more and more heavy and relaxed....

(Repeat)

'Think about your thigh muscles ... Tense them by pushing the tops of your legs together as hard as you can ... Feel the tension building ... Hold it ... Now, let your legs fall apart ... Feel the difference ... Feel the tension draining away from your legs ... They feel limp and heavy ... Your thighs feel heavy ... Your calves feel heavy ... Your feet feel heavy ... Imagine the tension draining away ... Leaving your legs ... Leaving them feeling limp and relaxed ... Leaving them feeling so heavy that they are sinking into the floor or your chair ... Let the feelings of relaxation spread up from your feet ... Up through your legs ... Relaxing your hips and lower back....

(Repeat)

'Now tense the muscles of your hips and lower back by squeezing your buttocks together ... Arch your back, gently ... Feel the tension ... Hold the tension ... Now let it go ... Let your muscles relax ... Feel your spine supported again...Feel the muscles relax ... Deeper and deeper ... More and more relaxed ... Growing heavier and heavier ... Your hips are relaxed ... Your legs are relaxed ... Your feet are heavy ... Tension is draining away from your body....

(Repeat)

'Tense your stomach and chest muscles, imagine that you are expecting a punch in the stomach and prepare yourself for the impact ... Take in a breath, and as you do, pull in your stomach and feel the muscles tighten ... Feel your chest muscles tighten and become rigid ... Hold the tension ... Now slowly breathe out and let go of the tension ... Feel your stomach muscles relax ... Feel the tightness leave your chest ... As you breathe evenly and calmly, your chest and stomach should gently rise and fall … Allow your breathing to become rhythmic and relaxed….

(Repeat)

'Now think about your hands and arms … Slowly curl your fingers into a tight fist … Feel the tension … Now hold your arms straight out in front of you, still clenching your fists … Feel the tension in your hands, your forearms and your upper arms … Hold it … Now, let go … Gently drop your arms by your side and imagine the tension draining away from your arms … Leaving your upper arms … Leaving your forearms … Draining away from your hands … Your arms feel heavy and floppy … Your arms feel limp and relaxed….

(Repeat)

'Think about the muscles in your shoulders … Tense them by drawing up your shoulders towards your ears and pull them in towards your spine … Feel the tension across your shoulders and in your neck … Tense the muscles in your neck further by tipping your head back slightly … Hold the tension … Now relax … Let your head drop forward … Let your shoulders drop … Let them drop even further … Feel the tension easing away from your neck and shoulders … Feel your muscles relaxing more and more deeply … Your neck is limp and your shoulders feel heavy….

(Repeat)

'Think about your face muscles … Focus on the muscles running across your forehead … Tense them by frowning as hard as you can … Hold that tension and focus on your jaw muscles … Tense the muscles by biting hard … Feel your jaw muscles tighten … Feel the tension in your face … Across your forehead … Behind your eyes … In your jaw … Now let go … Relax your forehead and drop your jaw … Feel the strain easing … Feel the tension draining away from your face … Your forehead feels smooth and relaxed … Your jaw is heavy and loose … Imagine the tension leaving your face … Leaving your neck … Draining away from your shoulders … Your head, neck, and shoulders feel heavy and relaxed….

(Repeat)

'Think of your whole body now … Your entire body feels heavy and relaxed … Let go of any tension … Imaging the tension flowing out of your body … Listen to the sound of your calm, even breathing … Your arms, legs, and head feel pleasantly heavy … Too heavy to move … You may feel as though you are floating … Don't be disturbed by this … Let it happen … It is part of being relaxed….

'When images drift into your mind, don't fight them … Just acknowledge them and let them pass … You are a bystander—interested but not involved … Enjoy the feelings of relaxation for a few more moments … If you like, picture something which gives you pleasure and a sense of calm….

'In a moment, I will count backwards from four to one … When I reach one, I want you to open your eyes and lie still for a little while before you begin to move around again … You will feel pleasantly relaxed and refreshed … Four: beginning to feel more alert … Three: getting ready to start moving again … Two: aware of your surroundings … One: eyes open, feeling relaxed and alert.'

Exercise 2: Shortened progressive relaxation or quick relaxation

'Now you can use the first exercise successfully, we can begin to shorten the routine by missing out the tensing stage. As you get better at this new routine, you can start to adapt it to use in different places at different times. Let's start the exercise by getting comfortable. Sit upright and well back into your chair, so that your thighs and back are supported. Rest your hands on your lap or on the arms of the chair and let your feet rest on the floor just beneath your knees.

'When you are sitting comfortably, close your eyes and let yourself unwind … Breathe out … Then breathe in as much as you need … Keep breathing rhythmically and slowly and deeply, relaxing a bit more with each breath … Feel the tension begin to ease away as you breathe out … You are now beginning to relax more deeply … Breathe out slowly … Breathe in smoothly and deeply … Now, breathe out slowly again, imagining yourself getting more and more heavy, sinking into your chair … Keep breathing rhythmically, and feel a sense of relief and of letting go … Try saying "relax" to yourself as you breathe out … Breathe like this for a few moments more….

'Now, we are going to relax all the muscles of your body … Think of your feet … Let your feet go limp and floppy … Feel the tension draining away from your feet ... Let your feet roll outwards and grow heavier and heavier ... Imagine that they are so heavy that they are sinking into the floor ... More and more relaxed ... Growing heavier and more relaxed....

'Now, think about your calves ... Imagine your leg muscles becoming floppy and heavy ... Feel the tension leaving your legs, draining from your calves ... Leaving your calves feeling heavy ... Draining away from your feet ... Leaving them feeling heavy and limp ... Imagine that your legs and feet are so heavy that they are sinking into the floor ... They feel limp and relaxed ... Growing more and more heavy and relaxed....

'Think about your thigh muscles ... Now, let your legs fall apart, limply ... Imagine the tension draining away from your legs ... They feel limp and heavy ... Your thighs feel heavy ... Your calves feel heavy ... Your feet feel heavy ... Imagine the tension draining away ... Leaving your legs ... Leaving them feeling limp and relaxed ... Leaving them feeling so heavy that they are sinking into the floor or your chair ... Let the feelings of relaxation spread up from your feet ... Up through your legs ... Relaxing your hips and lower back....

'Focus on the muscles of your hips and lower back ... Let go of any tension ... Let your muscles relax ... Feel your spine supported by your chair ... Feel the muscles relax ... Deeper and deeper ... More and more relaxed ... Growing heavier and heavier ... Your hips are relaxed ... Your legs are relaxed ... Your feet are heavy ... Tension is draining away from your body....

'Think of your stomach and chest muscles, and then slowly breathe out and let go of any tension ... Feel your stomach muscles relax ... Feel any tightness leave your chest ... As you breathe evenly and calmly, your chest and stomach should gently rise and fall ... Allow your breathing to become rhythmic and relaxed....

'Now think about your hands and arms ... Drop your arms by your side and imagine the tension draining away from your arms ... Leaving your upper arms ... Leaving your forearms ... Draining away from your hands ... Your arms feel heavy and floppy ... Your arms feel limp and relaxed....

'Think about the muscles in your shoulders and in your neck ... Let your head drop forward ... Let your shoulders drop ... Let them drop even further ... Feel any tension easing away from your neck and shoulders ... Feel your muscles relaxing more and more deeply ... Your neck is limp and your shoulders feel heavy....

'Now, think about the muscles in your face ... Let go of any tension ... Relax your forehead and drop your jaw ... Feel any strain easing ... All the tension draining away from your face ... Your forehead feels smooth and relaxed ... Your jaw is heavy and loose ... Imagine the tension leaving your face ... Leaving your neck ... Draining away from your shoulders ... Your head, neck, and shoulders feel heavy and relaxed....

'Think of your whole body, now ... Your entire body feels heavy and relaxed ... Let go of any tension ... Imagine it flowing out of your body ... Listen to the sound of your calm, even breathing ... Your arms, legs, and head feel pleasantly heavy ... Too heavy to move ... You may feel as though you are floating ... Don't be disturbed by this ... Let it happen ... It is part of being relaxed....

'When images drift into your mind, don't fight them ... Just acknowledge them and let them pass ... You are a bystander—interested but not involved ... Enjoy the feelings of relaxation for a few more moments ... If you like, picture something which gives you pleasure and a sense of calm....

'Soon, I will count backwards from four to one ... When I reach one, I want to open your eyes and lie still for a few more moments, before you begin to move around again ... You will feel pleasantly relaxed and refreshed ... Four: beginning to feel more alert ... Three: getting ready to start moving again ... Two: aware of your surroundings ... One: eyes open, feeling relaxed and alert.'

Exercise 3: Simple relaxation routine

'We can now go on to an even shorter exercise, which you can practise at almost any time you need to . For the shorter routine, you will need to imagine a mental image or mental device to use during the relaxation exercise. This can be a pleasant, calming scene, such as a deserted beach; a particularly relaxing picture or object; or sound or word which you find soothing, like the sound of the sea or the word "serene''. The important thing is that you should find a mental device which is calming for you.

'When you are doing this exercise, don't worry about how well you are performing—keep a passive attitude and allow the relaxation to work for you. Simply go at your own pace and don't try to force relaxation.

'With practice, this relaxation response will come with very little effort. You will then be able to respond to stress by relaxing almost automatically. In order to do this, however, you need to practise regularly.

'From time to time, distracting thoughts will come into your mind—this is quite usual. Don't dwell on them, simply return to thinking about your soothing image or sound. Once you have started the exercise, carry on for 10 or 20 minutes and, when you have finished, sit quietly with your eyes closed for a few moments. When you open your eyes, don't begin moving around too quickly.

'To start the exercise, sit in a comfortable position. First, focus on your breathing. Take a slow, deep breath in ... Feel the muscle beneath your rib cage move ... Now let it out—slowly ... Aim for a smooth pattern of breathing....

'Now, close your eyes, and, while you continue to breathe slowly, imagine your body becoming more heavy ... Scan your body for tension ... Start at your feet and move up through your body to your shoulders and head ... If you find any tension, try to relax that part of your body ... Now, while your body is feeling as heavy and comfortable as possible, become aware of your breathing again ... Breathe in through your nose, and fill your lungs fully ... Now, breathe out again and bring to mind your tranquil image or sound ... Breathe easily and naturally as you do this ... Again, breathe in through your nose, filling your lungs ... and out, thinking of your soothing mental device ... When you are ready to breathe in again, repeat the cycle ... Keep repeating this cycle until you feel relaxed and calm and refreshed.

'When you have finished this exercise, sit quietly for a few moments, and enjoy the feeling of relaxation.'

Appendix 7: *Some examples of diaries*

Diary 1

Anxiety record

Note down all the occasions when you experienced anxiety. Note them immediately after they happen or, if this is not possible, at the end of the day. *Do not leave it more than a day*. Rate your anxiety on each occasion on the following scale:

0	1	2	3	4	5	6	7	8	9	10
No anxiety really calm					Moderate anxiety					Absolute panic, worst possible

Record what brought on the anxiety (in terms of thoughts or fantasies, or specific events or situations) and what you did in response. Then re-rate your level of anxiety.

Date, time	Describe the occasion when you experienced the anxiety	Rating (0–10)	What brought about the anxiety—thoughts, events	What did you do?	Rating now (0–10)

Please bring this to your next appointment

Diary 2

Daily thought record

Note down all the occasions when you experienced anxiety. Note this immediately after they happen or, if this is not possible, at the end of the day. *Do not leave it for longer than a day*. Rate your anxiety on the following scale:

0	1	2	3	4	5	6	7	8	9	10
No anxiety really calm					Moderate anxiety					Absolute panic, worst possible

Then record what went through your mind when you felt anxious. After you have done this, think how you now might respond to your worrying thoughts in a rational, but not critical way. Then re-rate your anxiety level.

Date, time rating (0–10)	Situation: what were you doing?	Immediate thoughts: what exactly were your thoughts	Rational response: what were your rational answers to the thoughts	Rating now (0–10)

Please bring this to your next session. Thank you.

Diary 3

Symptom record

Note down all the occasions when you experienced unpleasant physical symptoms. Note them as they happen or, if this is not possible, at the end of the day. *Do not leave it more than a day*. Rate the severity on each occasion on the following scale:

0	1	2	3	4	5	6	7	8	9	10
No unpleasant physical experience(s)					Moderate level of unpleasant physical experience(s)					Very high level of unpleasant physical experience(s), worst ever

Record what was happening at the time (in terms of thoughts or fantasies, or specific events or situations) and what you did in response. Then re-rate the severity of your symptoms.

Date, time	Describe the occasion when you experienced the symptom(s)	Rating (0–10)	What brought about the symptom(s)—thoughts, events	What did you do?	Rating now (0–10)

Please bring this to your next session. Thank you.

Diary 4

Sleep Record

Record the date and note any events which might affect your sleep: e.g. what food you ate before going to bed, your stress levels, what exercise you took, etc. If you wake, note what you did to get back to sleep and whether or not this was helpful. Next day, note how many hours sleep you had and rate your levels of alertness (Rating 1) and how well you performed at your work (Rating 2), using the following scales.

1. Level of Alertness

1	2	3	4	5	6	7	8	9	10
Not alert				Quite alert					Very alert

2. Level of Performance

1	2	3	4	5	6	7	8	9	10
Poor performance				Reasonable					Performed well

Date	Notes—Food, stress, etc	Waking episodes	Activity if not sleep—helpful Y/N	Hours sleep	Rating 1	Rating 2

Appendix 8: *Book list and useful addresses*

Book List

Burns, D. (1990). *The feeling good handbook*. Plume, New York.

* Butler, G. (1985). *Managing anxiety*. Oxford University Press.

* Butler, G. (1992). *Managing social anxiety*. Oxford University Press.

Charlesworth, E. A. and Nathan, R. G. (1987). *Stress management*. Corgi Books, London.

Dickson, A. (1982). *A woman in your own right*. Quartet,

Haddon, C. (1984). *Women and tranquillisers*. Sheldon Press, London.

Hambly, K. (1983). *Overcoming tension*. Sheldon Press, London.

Jacobsen, E. (1976). *You must relax*. Souvenir Press, London.

Lindenfield, G. (1986). *Assert yourself*. Thorsons,

Madders, J. (1979). *Stress and relaxation*. Martin Dunitz, Cambridge.

Merrett, C. (1982). *Relaxation rules*. Minds Eye Books, Southsea.

Merrett, C. (1982). *Why worry*. Minds Eye Books, Southsea.

Mills, J. W. (1982). *Coping with stress*. Wiley Press, New York.

Smith, M. (1975). *When I say no, I feel guilty*. Bantam,

Trickett, S. A. *Coming off tranquillisers*. Sheldon Press, London.

Tyrer, P. (1980). *Stress: why it happens and how to overcome it*. Sheldon Press, London.

Weeks, C. (1976). *Self-help for your nerves*. Angus & Robertson, London.

Well Being Productions (1982). *Well being: helping yourself to health*. Penguin, Harmondsworth.

*Available from the Department of Psychology, Warneford Hospital, Oxford OX3 7JX.

Addresses

MIND
(National Association for Mental Health)
Granta House
15–19 Broadway
Stratford
London
E15 4BQ
0181 519 2122
Advice and information service on mental health problems.

The Open Door Association
447 Pensby Road
Heswall
Wirral
Merseyside
LR1 9PQ
Tel: 0151 443 0183
Information service for those with agoraphobia and anxiety states.

The Phobics Society
4 Cheltenham Road
Chorlton-cum-Hardy
Manchester
M21 1QN
Tel: 0161 881 1937
Self-help network of groups to help phobics with everyday problems.

Relaxation for Living
168–170 Oatlands Drive
Weybridge
Surrey
KT13 9ET
Tel: 0932 831000
Promotes relaxation to combat anxiety and tension. Teachers run classes around the country and also a correspondence course. Leaflets and cassettes available.

Release
388 Old Street
London
EC1 9LT
Tel: 0171 729 9904
Advice and information on drug use and abuse.

Stresswatch
PO Box 4
London
W1A 4AR
Organization to help those with phobic and anxiety states. Postal advice and weekend workshop and cassettes available.

References

American Psychiatric Association (1980). *Diagnostic and statistical manual of mental disorders* (3rd. ed.) Washington DC.

Ashton, C. H. (1984). Benzodiazepine withdrawal: an unfinished story. *British Medical Journal*, **228**, 1135–40.

Atkinson, R. M., Sparr, L. F., Sheff, A. G., White, R., and Fitzsimmons, J. T. (1984). Diagnosis of PTSD in Vietnam veterans: preliminary findings. *American Journal of Psychiatry*, **141**, 694–6.

Bandura, A. (1970). *Principles of behaviour modification*. Holt, Rinehart & Winston, London.

Barker, C., Pistrang, N., Shapiro, D. A. and Shaw, I. (1990). Coping and help seeking in the UK adult population. *British Journal of Clinical Psychology*, **29**, 271–85.

Beck, A. T., Emery, G., and Greenberg, R. (1985). *Anxiety disorders and phobias: a cognitive perspective*. Basic Books, New York.

Beck, A. T., Rush, A. J., Shaw, B. F., and Emery, G. (1979). *Cognitive therapy of depression*. The Guildford Press, New York.

Beck, A. T., Brown, G., and Steer, R. A. (1986). Beck Anxiety Check-list. Unpublished manuscript, Centre for Cognitive Therapy.

Benson, H. (1975). *The relaxation response*. Collins Fount Publications, Glasgow.

Butler, G. (1985). *Managing anxiety*. Hall the Printer, Oxford.

Carlson, N. R. (1977). The nature and function of sleep. In: *Physiology of behaviour*, pp. 338–409. Allyn and Bacon Inc, Boston.

Catalan, J. and Gath, D. (1985). Benzodiazepines in general practice: a time for decision. *British Medical Journal*, **290**, 375–6.

Catalan, J., Gath, D., Edmonds, G., and Ennis, J. (1984). The effects of non-prescribing of anxiolytics in general practice. *British Journal of Psychiatry*, **144**, 593–602.

Clark, D. M. (1987). A cognitive approach to panic: theory and data. Paper presented at the 140th annual meeting of the American Psychiatric Association, Chicago.

Clark, D. M., Salkovskis, P. M., and Chalkley, A. J. (1985). Respiratory control as a treatment for panic attacks. *Journal of Behaviour Therapy and Experimental Psychiatry*, **16**, No. 1, 23–30.

Committee on the Review of Medicines. (1980). Systematic review of benzodiazepines. *British Medical Journal*, **i**, 910–12.

Cooper, B. (1979). Clinical and social aspects of chronic neurosis: Proceedings of the Royal Society of Medicine (1972). In: *Psychosocial disorders in general practice* (ed. P. Williams and A. Clare). Academic Press, London.

Cowell McFarlane, A. (1988). The aetiology of PTSD following a natural disaster. *British Journal of Psychiatry*, **152**, 116–21.

Dement, W. C. (1972). *Some must watch while some must sleep*. W. H. Freeman & Co, San Francisco.

Driver, H. S. and Shapiro, C. M. (1993). Parasomnias. *British Medical Journal*, **306**, 921–4.

D'Zurilla, T. and Nezu, A. (1982). Social problem solving in adults. In *Advances in cognitive-behavioural research and therapy* (ed. D. Kendall), Vol. 1. Academic Press, New York).

Ellis, A. (1962). *Reason and emotion in psychotherapy*. Lyle Stuart, New York.

Finlay-Jones, R. and Brown, G. W. (1981). Types of stressful events and the onset of anxiety and depressive disorders. *Psychological Medicine*, **11**, 803–15.

Freud, S., Ferenczi, S., Abraham, K., Simmel, E., and Jones, E. (1921). *Psychoanalysis and the war neurosis*. International Psychoanalytic Press, New York.

Freud, S. (1926). On psychopathology: Inhibitions, symptoms and anxiety. In *The Pelican Freud Library* (ed. A. Richards), Vol. 10. (1979). Penguin Books, Middlesex.

Freudenberger, H. J. (1974). Staff burn-out. *Journal of Social Issues*, **30**, 159–65.

Gelder, M. G. (1985). Psychological treatments for anxiety disorders. Paper given to the University Department of Psychiatry, Oxford.

Gelder, M. G., Gath, D. H., and Mayou, R. (1989). *The Oxford textbook of psychiatry* (second edition). Oxford University Press.

Goldberg, D. and Huxley, P. (1980). *Mental illness in the community: the pathway to psychiatric care*. Tavistock Publications, London.

Goldfried, M. and Davidson, G. (1976). *Clinical behaviour therapy*. Holt, Rinehart & Winston, New York.

Higgitt, A. C., Lader, M. H., and Fonagy, P. (1985). Clinical management of benzodiazepine dependence. *British Medical Journal*, **291**, 668–90.

Jacobsen, E. (1983). *Progressive relaxation*. University of Chicago Press.

Kales, A., Soldatos, C. R., Bixler, E. O., and Kales, J. D. (1983). Rebound insomnia and rebound anxiety. *Pharmacology*, **26**, 121–37.

Kazdin, A. E. (1974). Reactive self-monitoring: the effects of response desirability, goal setting and feedback. *Journal of Consulting and Clinical Psychology*, **42**, 704–16.

Kinzie, J. D., Fredrickson, R. H., Ben, R., Flick, J., and Karls, W. (1984). PTSD among survivors of Cambodian concentration camps. *American Journal of Psychiatry*, **141**, 645–50.

Lacey, R. and Woodward, S. (1985) *That's Life survey on tranquillisers*. BBC publications in association with MIND, London.

Lader, M. H. (1992). Guidelines for the management of patients with generalized anxiety. *Bulletin of the Royal Colleges of Psychiatry*, **16**, 560–5.

Lader, M. H. (1984). Working out a withdrawal plan. In *Women and tranquillisers* (ed. C. Hadden), pp. 69–72. Sheldon Press, London.

Lancet (1979). Editorial, Part 1. *Lancet*, **1**, 478–9.

Loughrey, G. C., Bell, P., Kee, M., Roddy, R. J., and Curran, P. S. (1988). PTSD and civil violence in Northern Ireland. *British Journal of Psychiatry*, **153**, 554–60.

McCue, E. C. and McCue, P. A. (1984). Organic and hyperventilatory causes of anxiety-type symptoms. *British Association for Behavioural Psychotherapy*, **12**, 308–17.

McPherson, I. G. (1981). Clinical psychology in primary health care. In: *Reconstructing clinical practice*, (ed. I. G. McPherson and A. Sutton), pp. 21–41. Croom Helm, London.

Marks, I. M. (1985). A controlled trial of psychiatric nurse therapists in primary care. *British Medical Journal*, **290**, 1181–4.

Marks, I. M. (1987). *Fears, phobias and rituals: panic, anxiety and their disorders*. Oxford University Press.

Marks, I. M. (1991). Self-administered behavioural treatment. *Behavioural Psychotherapy*, **19**, 42–6.

Maslach, C. and Pines, A. (1979). Burnout: the loss of human caring. In *Experiencing social psychology*. (ed. C. Maslach). Random House, New York.

Meichenbaum, D. (1971). Examination of model characteristics in reducing avoidance behaviour. *Journal of Personality and Social Psychology*, **17**, 298–307.

Meichenbaum, D. (1985). *Stress inoculation training*. Pergamon Press, Oxford.

Noyes, R., Crowe, P. R., Hoenk, P. R., and Slymen, D. J. (1978). The familial prevalence of anxiety neurosis. *Archives of General Psychiatry*, **35**, 1057–9.

Ost, L. G., Jerremalam, and A., Johansson, J. (1981). Individual response patterns and the effects of different behavioural methods in the treatment of social phobia. *Behaviour Research and Therapy*, **19**, 1–16.

Ost, L. G., Johansson, J., and Jerremalam, A. (1982). Individual response patterns and the effects of different behavioural methods in the treatment of claustrophobia. *Behaviour Research and Therapy*, **20**, 445–60.

Oswald, I. (1962). *Sleeping and waking: physiology and psychology*. Elsevier Publishing Company, Amsterdam.

Peveler, R., and Johnston, D. W. (1986). Subjective and cognitive effects of relaxation. *Behaviour Research and Therapy*, **24**, 413–20.

Rachman, S. (1966). Studies in desensitisation: III. Speed of generalisation. *Behavioural Research and Therapy*, **4**, 7.

Robinson, C. and Suinn, R. (1969). Group desensitisation of a phobia and massed sessions. *Journal of Behavioural Research and Therapy*, **7**, 319.

Rossenman, R. H., Friedman, M., and Straus, R. (1964). A predictive study of CHD. *Journal of the American Medical Association*, **195**, 86–92.

Rothbaum, B. O., Foa, E. B., Murdock, T., Riggs, D., and Walsh, W. (1990). PTSD in rape victims (unpublished manuscript).

Salkovskis, P. M., Jones, D. R. O., and Clark, D. M. (1986). Respiratory control in the treatment of panic attacks: relication. *British Journal of Psychiatry*, **13**, 526–32.

Schweizer, E. and Rickels, K. (1991). Pharmacotherapy of generalized anxiety disorder. In *Chronic anxiety, generalized anxiety disorder and mixed anxiety and depression*. (ed. R. M. Rapee and D. H. Barlow), pp. 172–86. Guilford Press, New York.

Sorby, N. G. D., Reavley, W., and Huber, J. W. (1991). Self-help programme for anxiety in general practice: controlled trial of an anxiety management booklet. *British Journal of General Practice*, **41**, 417–20.

Speilberger, C. D., Gorsuch, R. L., Lushene, R., Vagg, P. R., and Jacobs, G. A. (1983). *The manual for the state-trait anxiety inventory*. Consulting Psychologist Press Inc., Palo Alto, CA.

Stradling, J. R. (1993). Recreational drugs and sleep. *British Medical Journal*, **306**, 573–5.

Suinn, R. M. and Richardson, F. (1971). Anxiety management training: A non-specific behaviour therapy programme for anxiety control. *Behaviour Therapy*, **2**, 498–510.

Telch, M. J., Lucas, J. A., Schmidt, N. B., Hanna, H. H., LaNaeJaimez, T., Luca, R. A. (1993). Group cognitive–behavioural treatment of panic disorder. *Behavoural Research and Therapy*, **31**, 279–87.

Tyrer, P. J. (1984). Benzodiazepines on trial. *British Medical Journal*, **288**, 1101–2.

Tyrer, P. J. and Murphy, S. (1987). The place of benzodiazepines in psychiatric practice. *British Journal of Psychiatry*, **151**, 719–23.

Williams, T. (ed.) (1980). *Post-traumatic stress disorders of the Vietnam veteran.* Disabled American Veterans, Cincinnata, OH.

Wolpe, J. (1958). *Psychotherapy by reciprocal inhibition*. Stanford University Press, Stanford, CA.

Wolpe, J. (1985). *The practice of behavior therapy* (third edition). Pergamon Press, New York.

Index